EMERGENCY SERVICES CONTACTS

- **Royal Flying Doctor Service radio frequencies and telephone numbers—see page 00**
- **Ambulance Fire Police—call 000**
- **Satellite Phone—call short code 13 national operator transfer to emergency services**
- **Diver Emergency Service—call 1800 088 200 (within Australia) or +61 8 8373 5312 (from outside Australia)**
- **Poisons Information Centre—call 13 11 26**
- **HF radio frequency—range 2–30 MHz, or 2–6 MHz**
- **UHF/CB radio—channel 5 for emergency transmission**

Clearly identify your location (give map and grid references), and number and condition of casualties.

The information and numbers above were correct at the time of publication.

Australian Remote Area First Aid

St John Ambulance Australia

St John Ambulance Australia
Canberra Avenue
FORREST ACT 2603

First published in 1991 as *Survival! Remote Area First Aid*
New edition 2000

ISBN 0 949569 44 5

Editors: Shirley Dyson, Vic Groenhout
Writers: Alan Caust, Robert Correa, Alan Stewart, Cass Tucker
Designer: Goro Jankulovski
Photographer: Chris Groenhout
Illustrator: Dr Levent Efe
Production Management: Acute Image Pty Ltd
Copyedit: Perfect Words

Typeset in Palatino

Colour separation and reproduction by Impact Printing (Melbourne)

Printed and bound by Impact Printing (Melbourne)

Contents

Acknowledgments

St John Ambulance Australia would like to thank those who contributed to the development of 'Australian Remote Area First Aid'. In particular, the organisation thanks the following groups and individuals for their support:

St John Ambulance Australia Training Centres

St John Ambulance Service, Northern Territory

Czeslawa Markiewicz, Andrew Kentler, Tom Wain, Joan Schneider, Michael Carver, Mari Jankulovska, Pavlina Siljanovska, Steve Nackovski, Steve Peers, Grant Stowell, Mark Todoroski, Trent Nankervis, Gabriela Jankulovska, David White, Professor Michael O'Rourke, Dr Peter Sullivan, Dr Peter Warfe

Royal Flying Doctor Service, Air Ambulance Victoria, Victorian Police Air Wing, Metropolitan Ambulance Service (Victoria), Paddy Pallen (Melbourne), City Centre Disposals (Melbourne), Water Police (Melbourne), Police Search and Rescue (Melbourne), Asthma Victoria, Toyota Australia, Natural Resources & Environment, Dick Smith Electronics, Country Fire Authority, Victoria Ranges, Australian Maritime Safety Authority, Emergency Management Australia

Foreword

Almost ten years have passed since St John Ambulance Australia first published this book's predecessor *Survival! Remote Area First Aid*. In that time there have been great advances in communications technology. Devices such as mobile phones, Global Positioning Systems (GPS), electronic distress beacons (EPIRBs) and the Internet have changed the very concept of remoteness—providing new methods by which people can call for assistance or summon-up information. However, technological advance is still no substitute for knowledge, skill and compassion in dealing with sick or injured casualties in an isolated setting.

The Wilderness Medical Society defines wilderness as 'a remote geographical location more than one hour from definitive medical care'. Accepting that definition, this book is highly relevant not only to those who live and work on farms or other remote and rural locations throughout Australia, but to the increasing number of people who enjoy outdoor leisure activities such as bushwalking, skiing, camping, four-wheel driving, fishing, climbing, sailing, kayaking and a host of other adventurous pursuits.

Australian Remote Area First Aid has been designed to help you acquire knowledge so that you may ease pain and save lives. But real-life experience will quickly demonstrate that wilderness or remote area first aid rarely allows for recipe-book solutions that will cover every situation. Such limitations on what actually can be achieved in a remote setting provide another good reason why this book quite rightly stresses planning, preparation and prevention.

St John Ambulance Australia has a long and proud tradition of providing first aid care to the public, and of teaching practical life-saving skills to a significant portion of the Australian population. This book is one more step in achieving the St John Ambulance mission of 'Caring for Life in the Community', in even the most remote corners of our nation.

Dr Peter Sullivan
Medical Research Officer, Australian Antarctic Division

Introduction

Even before my transition—more than three decades ago—from city nurse to bush bird living in extreme isolation, I believed that first aid should be a compulsory component of every school curriculum. My subsequent experiences on our remote cattle station, situated 600 km south west of Katherine in the Northern Territory, have reinforced that conviction. Knowledge and understanding instilled in young minds become part of one's psyche. The resultant ability and confidence to put theory into practice is then more likely to become automatic. Of course, basic principles and management practices require regular review.

Given the recognition of the need for urban dwellers to have adequate first aid knowledge and skills, consider the situation beyond the familiar and reassuring community infrastructure. Our magnificent, timeless inland shows no mercy to the foolish or ill-prepared. Remote Australia, in all its wonder and glory, commands respect from inhabitants and visitors alike.

Be aware that in the land of the unknown there is always the unexpected. Do not let the overwhelming sense of freedom associated with the splendour of never-ending horizons distract you from the critical need for preparedness, planning and accountability. Remember the golden rule of the bush: always advise someone somewhere of your departure point and estimated time of arrival at your destination.

As the magical lure of the outback and the unexplored touches more and more lives, on a local, national and international level, it is timely to prioritise preparation for visiting a remote area. The physical and practical check lists are widely identified; however, equally critical are first aid kits combined with the necessary skills, communication options and the all-important ability to manage a casualty for an extended period of time as necessary until medical assistance arrives.

This *Australian Remote Area First Aid* book should become every traveller's bible. It rates pride of place in schoolbags, roadhouses, hotels, humpies, stock camps, homesteads and holiday resorts. It has an application for each and every one of us.

Terry Underwood (Mrs), Author
In the Middle of Nowhere
Riveren: My Home, Our Country

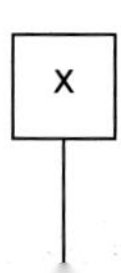
x

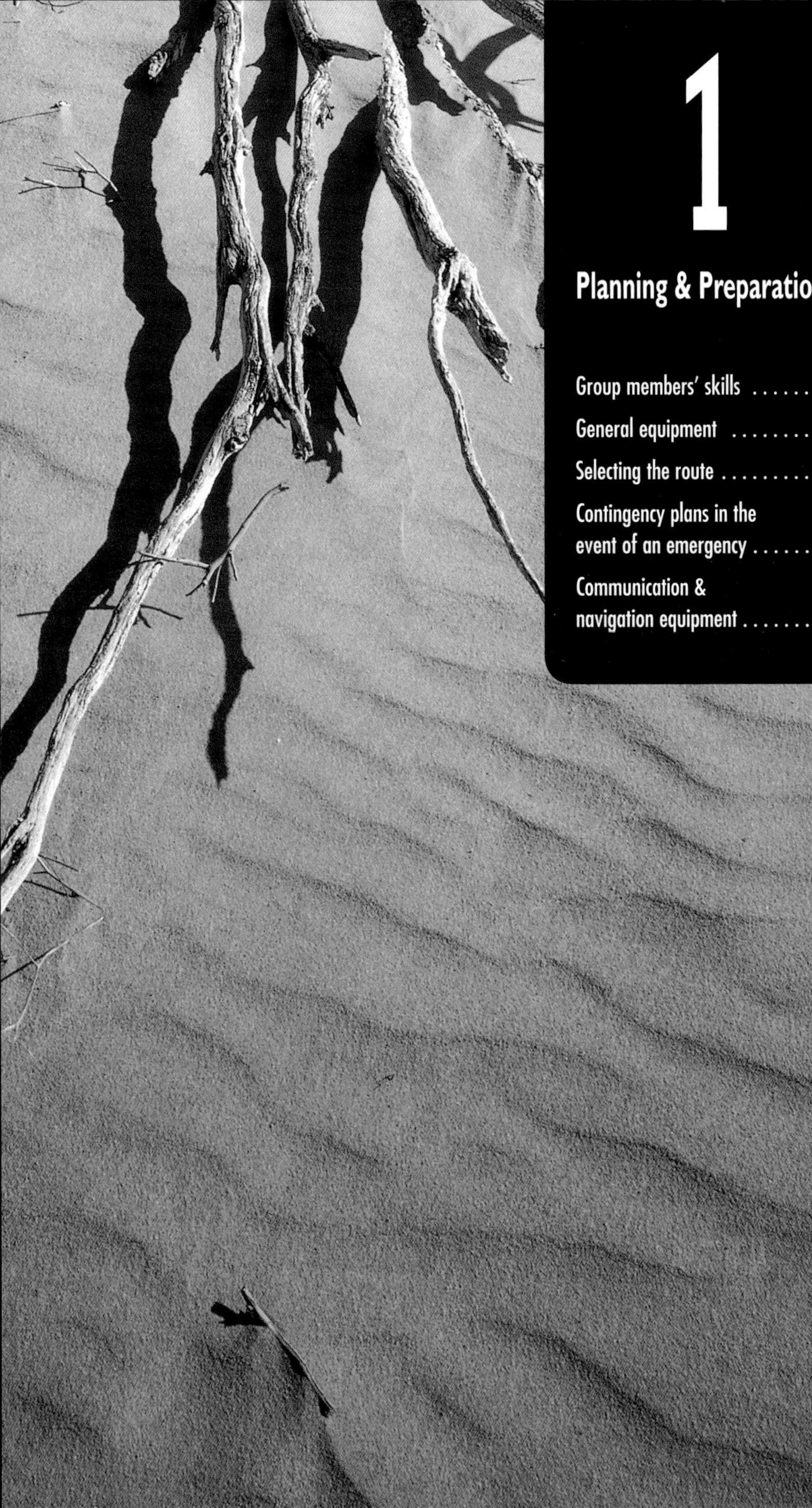

1

Planning & Preparation

In examining the journeys undertaken by explorers such as Sturt, in eastern Australia, and Mawson, in the Antarctic, you recognise that these journeys depended on the quality of planning and preparation. Most of us will not undertake—either for work or recreation—journeys as long, difficult or dangerous as those of Sturt and Mawson. However, the outoor activities we do undertake possess some of the characteristics of their journeys.

Outdoor adventure activities often involve small groups of people travelling into remote areas completely dependent on the resources of the group and the equipment carried. In the event of something going wrong they must be able to rely on their own resources at least for a period of time. The response to 'something going wrong' can in extreme cases literally make the difference between life and death. In less serious cases it may simply make the difference between a long, cold, uncomfortable night and a dry, comfortable one.

What must be considered is that being able to achieve what we set out to do, safely and with enjoyment, is not a matter of luck. It does not just 'happen'. It is, as it was for Sturt and Mawson, largely a reflection of the care taken in planning and preparation.

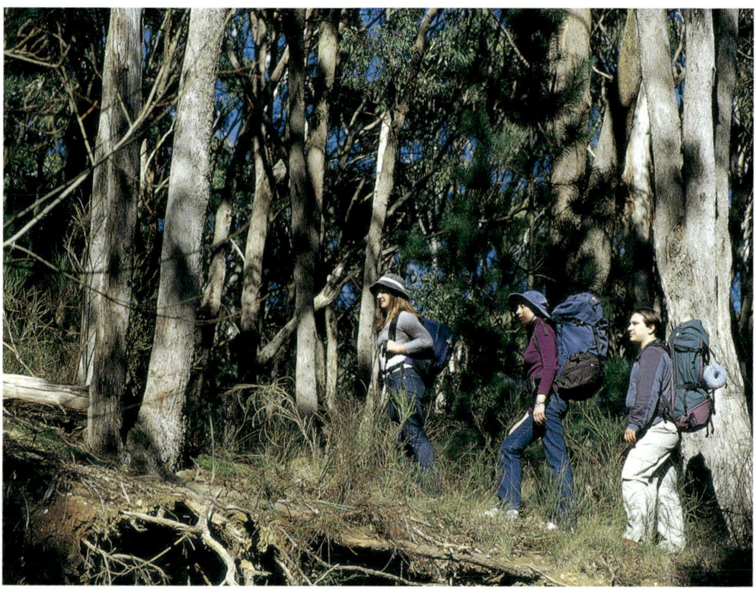

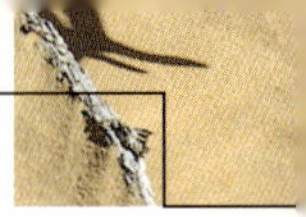

Planning and preparation are vital parts of any activity. In outdoor activities in which a group is dependent on its own resources, the importance of thorough planning and preparation cannot be overestimated. These factors can facilitate the group achieving their objectives safely.

In the planning and preparation phase of an outdoor activity, factors to consider include:

- group members' skills
- general equipment
- selecting the route
- contingency plan in the event of an emergency
- communication and navigation equipment

Group members' skills

Each member's levels of fitness, experience and skills need to be considered in relation to the planned activity. Does the individual possess the level of physical fitness the activity will demand? Do they have the experience and skills necessary to undertake the activity safely? These are questions that need to be considered carefully before the activity begins. Individuals whose fitness is not at the required level for the activity may place themselves and the group in potential danger.

For example a person who is struggling to keep up with the rest of the group and is progressively becoming more fatigued may not be able to continue. In the event of a severe deterioration in the weather or a miscalculation of the actual time needed to travel over the terrain, this situation could become dangerous for the individual and the group.

The same is true for the individual's level of experience and skill. While a person needs to participate in activities to gain experience and develop skills, it needs to be considered at the planning stage whether or not it is appropriate or safe for an inexperienced person to participate. For example, a person may be able to abseil a single pitch but their experience is limited to having completed a training course. Would it be appropriate or safe for them to participate in an activity involving a multiple pitch descent in possibly less than ideal conditions?

Essentially what needs to be considered: Is the group fit enough and do the members have the experience and skills to undertake the proposed activity? If, after careful consideration, the answer to this question is 'no' or 'perhaps not', then the scope of the activity needs to be reconsidered.

In any activity in which members of a small group have to rely on one another and, in an emergency, be absolutely dependent on one another, the specialist skills they have should be known by the group.

The awareness that some members are skilled in areas such as leadership, navigation, first aid and rescue may give others a greater degree of confidence and can facilitate the allocation of responsibility within the group. This allocation is an essential part of planning and preparation—for example, who will be group leader, first aider and navigator.

Further, as part of the planning process, it is important that the leader knows if any members of the group have a medical condition which may require medication. However, an individual's privacy must be considered. People should be encouraged to identify only those medical conditions which, in an emergency, could be life-threatening or which the individual's doctor considers risky for the planned activity. For example a person with asthma who wishes to pursue scuba diving should declare the condition because of the potential danger.

Any medical information disclosed to the leader or first aider must be considered confidential. It should only be disclosed if there is good reason, e.g. in an emergency involving the individual.

General equipment

In the planning and preparation phase the equipment required, including safety and emergency gear, food, fuel and clothing needs to be selected for the type of activity planned. While most activities require some equipment, there is no universal list of equipment for all purposes.

Each piece of equipment needs to be assessed in relation to its planned use. For example a tent which is ideal for warm weather camping is not necessarily suited to or safe for use in the snow.

The choice of appropriate **clothing, sleeping bag and shelter** can make a trip much more enjoyable. In deteriorating or poor weather, lack of suitable clothing and camping gear may make the situation life-threatening.

The **first aid kit** selected must be adequate for the type of activity planned and its duration.

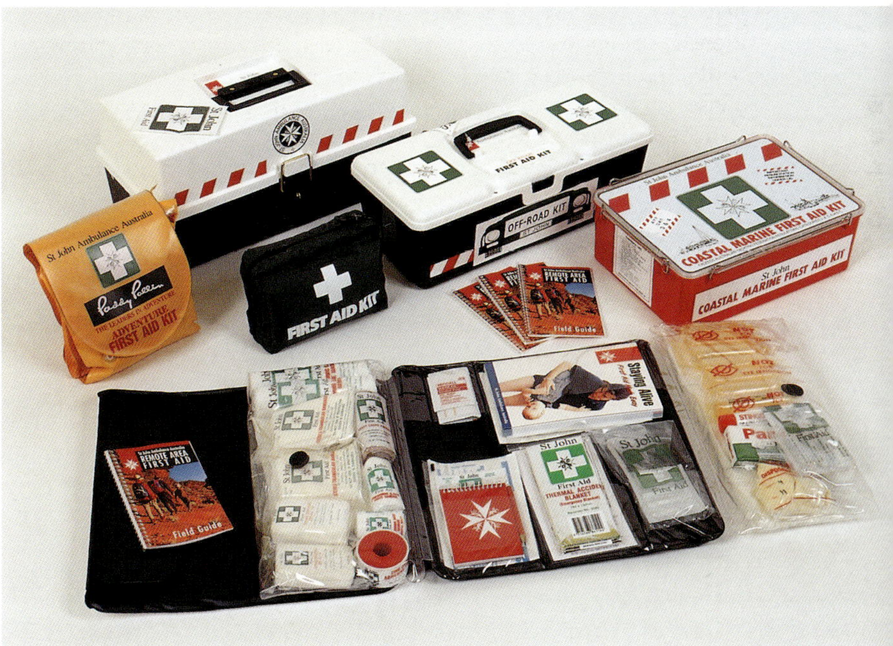

In many areas of Australia **fuel stoves** rather than wood fires need to be used for cooking. When travelling in these areas the volume of fuel carried needs to be sufficient to meet the food preparation needs of the group. Most stoves are reliable and safe to use but as with all equipment, knowledge of use and maintenance is necessary.

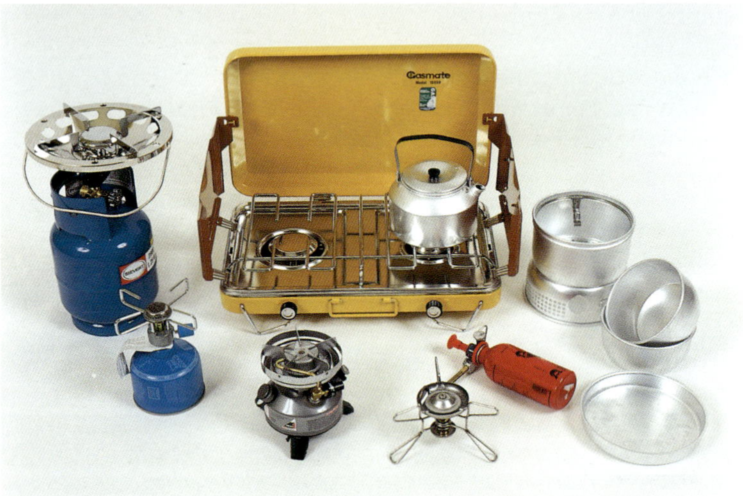

When selecting the **foods** to be taken on an activity, factors such as weight, bulk, ease of preparation, enjoyment and energy provided need to be considered. To reduce weight and bulk, dehydrated or freeze-dried foods are often selected. This type of food is quick and easy to prepare; however it does require access to adequate supplies of water to rehydrate the food.

In many areas, a lack of adequate **water** along the intended route can be a limiting factor, particularly for those travelling on foot. When touring, you will find that most towns have water but at some places you may not be able to get drinking water. It is better to carry your own drinking water, and not rely on a waterhole, dam, bore, mill, tank or trough as your source of water supply.

Most people need at least eight glasses of water a day to maintain an adequate level of hydration. If active—e.g. walking or climbing you will need additional water at regular intervals.

Remember: Don't wait to feel thirsty before you drink.

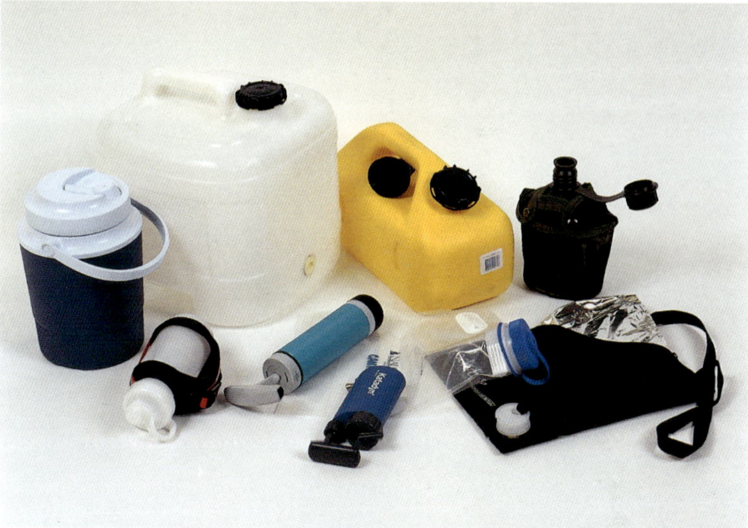

Various types of water containers and purifiers

On an overnight trip in extreme conditions, the inability to adequately replace energy and/or fluids may not only cause discomfort but also endanger the group. To function effectively, we need to replace fluid lost through sweating and consume food to provide energy.

Checking equipment

All equipment needs to be checked before setting out to ensure that it is in good condition and working correctly. Ensure that group members are trained in the use of all items of equipment. Trying to erect a tent that you are not familiar with can, even in good conditions, take time. In a storm it may take much longer.

Prior to the group departing on the activity, a kit/backpack check needs to be carried out to ensure that every member has the equipment required for the activity.

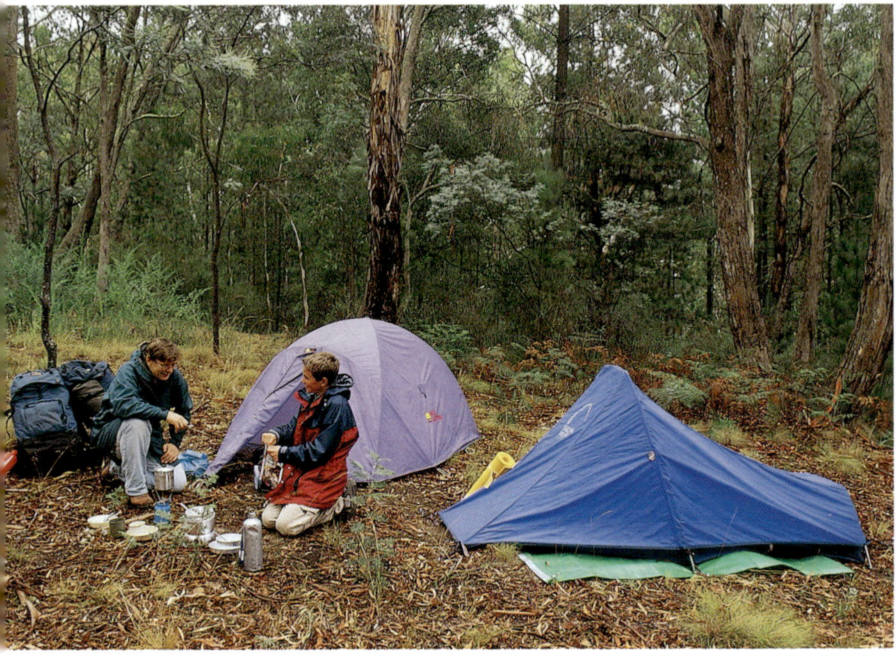

Selecting the route

In selecting a route the group can gain a great deal of information by studying the map(s) of the area, referring to any specific track notes, and by talking with those who know the area. The old adage 'time spent in reconnaissance is never wasted' is very true.

Alternative routes also need to be planned so that if it becomes necessary to shorten the activity and get the group out in the shortest time, e.g. due to bad weather or illness, that option will have been considered and a route determined.

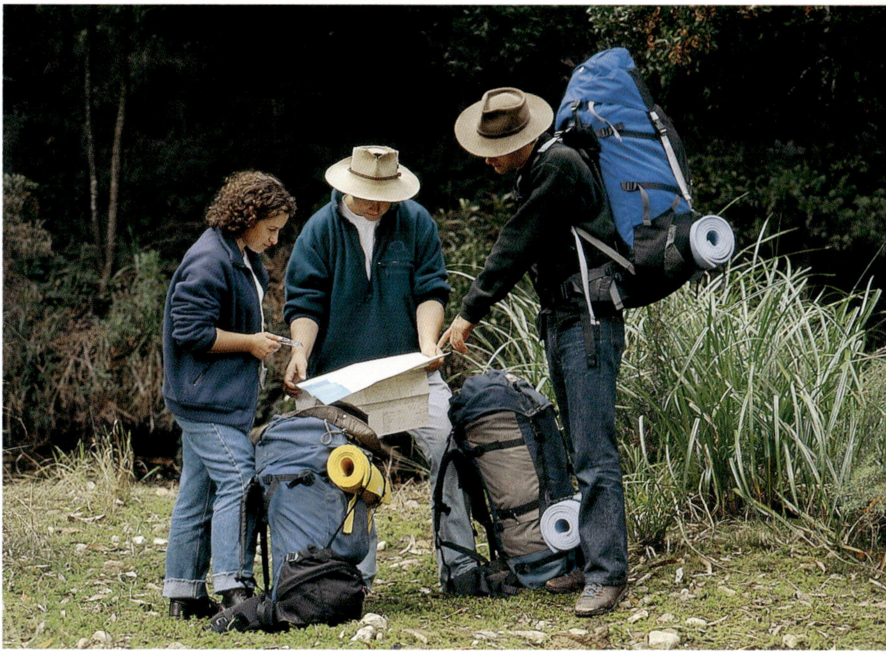

Once the route is selected, the group can then prepare a navigation data chart. This is done by identifying the starting point and selecting other key points along the route, which are identified by their respective grid references.

The bearings from one key point to the next can then be calculated using a compass and protractor. Distances from one bound to another can also be determined from the map. This data is then entered on a navigation data sheet as follows:

From	To Bearing	Magnetic in Metres	Distance Time	Estimated	Notes
970351	985398	286°	750 m	25 minutes	Cross creek at 500m then uphill

By preparing the navigation data sheet before commencing the activity, the navigational information is calculated and checked in optimal conditions. There is no wind blowing the map, cold fingers handling the protractor or tired eyes trying to scrutinise the map in failing light. The information, with clearly identified camp sites, should be made available to all group members.

Plans including routes and timings must always be given to either rangers, police, emergency services or friends/relations before commencing the activity.

Contingency plans in the event of an emergency

Contingency plans for possible emergencies should be considered by the group in the planning stage. For example, you may have contingency plans for a member becoming separated from the group, or being injured or ill and unable to continue.

The optimal time to consider what needs to be done and how to do it is at the planning stage, not at the time of the emergency when emotions can run high and the ability to make critical decisions is impaired. The safety of an individual or the group may depend on a definite plan having been formulated and communicated to all members so that they know what is expected of them in the situation.

Contingency plans need to be considered as a priority.

Lost or separated from group

If you become aware that you are separated from your group or that you are lost:

- stop, stay calm, do not continue on
- look around or use your map to try to establish where you are
- if you can positively identify where you are and can navigate back to your correct route, do so—your group members will be looking for you on or near the route
- if you are carrying a Global Positioning System *(see p. 14)* it will assist you in locating your position and the direction you are heading

If you cannot identify where you are:

- remain where you are and stay calm—attempt to indicate your position by:
  - calling out at frequent intervals
  - listening for calls being returned
  - blowing a whistle in a series of three
  - using mobile phone or radio—if signal is weak go to high ground

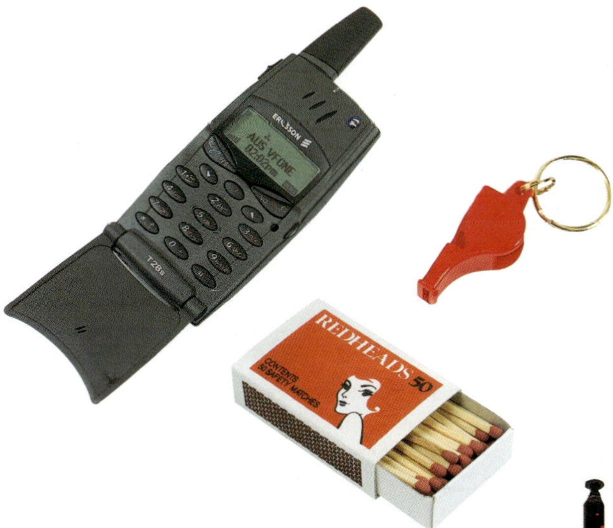

If your group cannot find you:

- activate Emergency Position Indicating Rescue Beacon (EPIRB) if available *(see p. 58)*
- establish camp, preferably in an open area visible from the air, or on a high point—this may not be possible in extreme conditions
- light a fire if safe to do so and make smoke—clear ground 3–4 metres radius around fire

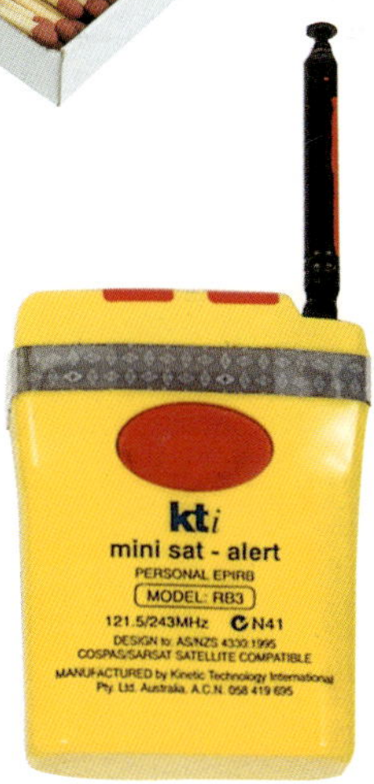

- during the day, lay out markers on the ground using sleeping bags, tent fly, groundsheet, boating V sheet; make marks or lay out rocks on the ground—the markers need to be large
- conserve energy, food and water

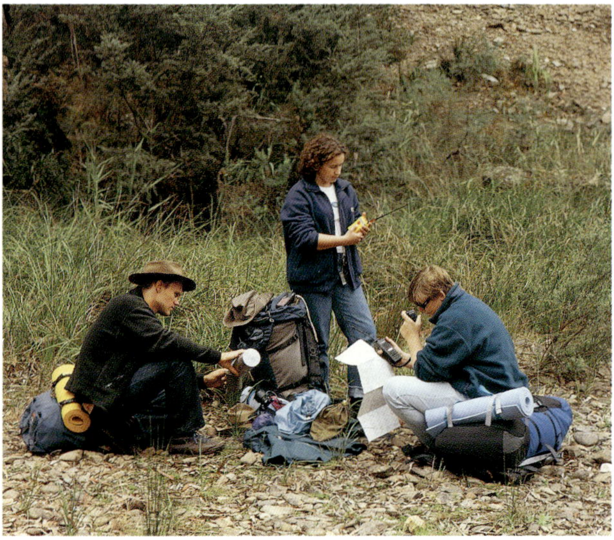

Member of group injured, ill or cannot continue

When an individual is seriously injured or ill, the actions taken by the group are determined by the need to assist the casualty, call for help and ensure the safety of the casualty until help arrives.

The decision not to continue the activity can be made more difficult when a member of a group, through fatigue, loss of confidence or minor injury, feels unable to continue. In this situation the remainder of the group may be anxious to continue on and as a result the group splits.

While it may be tempting to suggest that the individual who is unable to continue could rest and then either try to catch up with the group or make their own way out of the area, the potential risks of these options must be considered. The following questions need to be answered satisfactorily:

- can they manage to look after themselves until they recover?

- can they manage a severe change in the weather?
- can they find their way?
- do they have adequate equipment?

A plan in which the group goes in and comes out together is safer than one in which the group splits. When separated, a small group potentially loses the capabilities brought to it by the combined skills of its members.

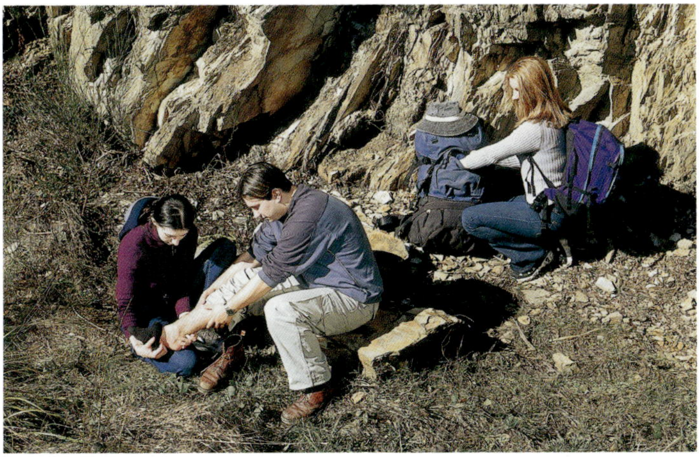

Group overdue on return time

Before departure, the group should leave with someone a route plan showing camp sites, any side trips and the latest date/time they expect to return. This person needs to be briefed to notify the police of these details if the group does not return on time.

Based on the level of experience of the group, the equipment carried and prevailing weather conditions, the police will determine if and when to commence a search. Information on the route can greatly assist any search and rescue activity.

Communication & navigation equipment

In the planning and preparation stage, the group will need to determine the most appropriate communication equipment for the area in which they are travelling. Mobile phones, satellite phones and radios give those entering remote areas the ability to call and receive help in a relatively short time. This provides a great deal of security and, in most situations, ensures that help can be obtained quickly.

In some situations, because of constraints imposed by the terrain, available space and the weight to be carried, the group may decide that, although voice communication is the optimum, they will instead carry an EPIRB.

Whatever system the group decides to use, they must be absolutely sure that it works effectively in the area in which they will be travelling.

Global Positioning System (GPS)

The pocket-sized and economical GPS is a powerful navigation tool that uses satellites to establish reference points from which to calculate positions accurate to a matter of metres. The GPS has eight keypad functions that operate a number of screens such as:

- satellite—shows satellite positions and signal strength
- position—shows where you are and the direction you are travelling
- map—allows you to view your position and surrounding waypoint symbols such as fuel, medical aid, lake etc.
- compass—has a rotating compass display to show your direction of travel and guide you to a destination; the compass screen provides guidance for car travel, hiking, or biking where straight-line navigation is usually not possible

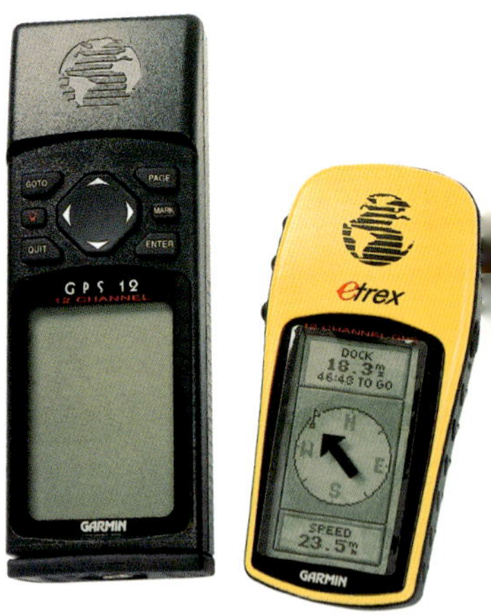

Note: If you choose to carry a GPS it is advisable to study the manual thoroughly and practise using the GPS prior to travelling in remote areas.

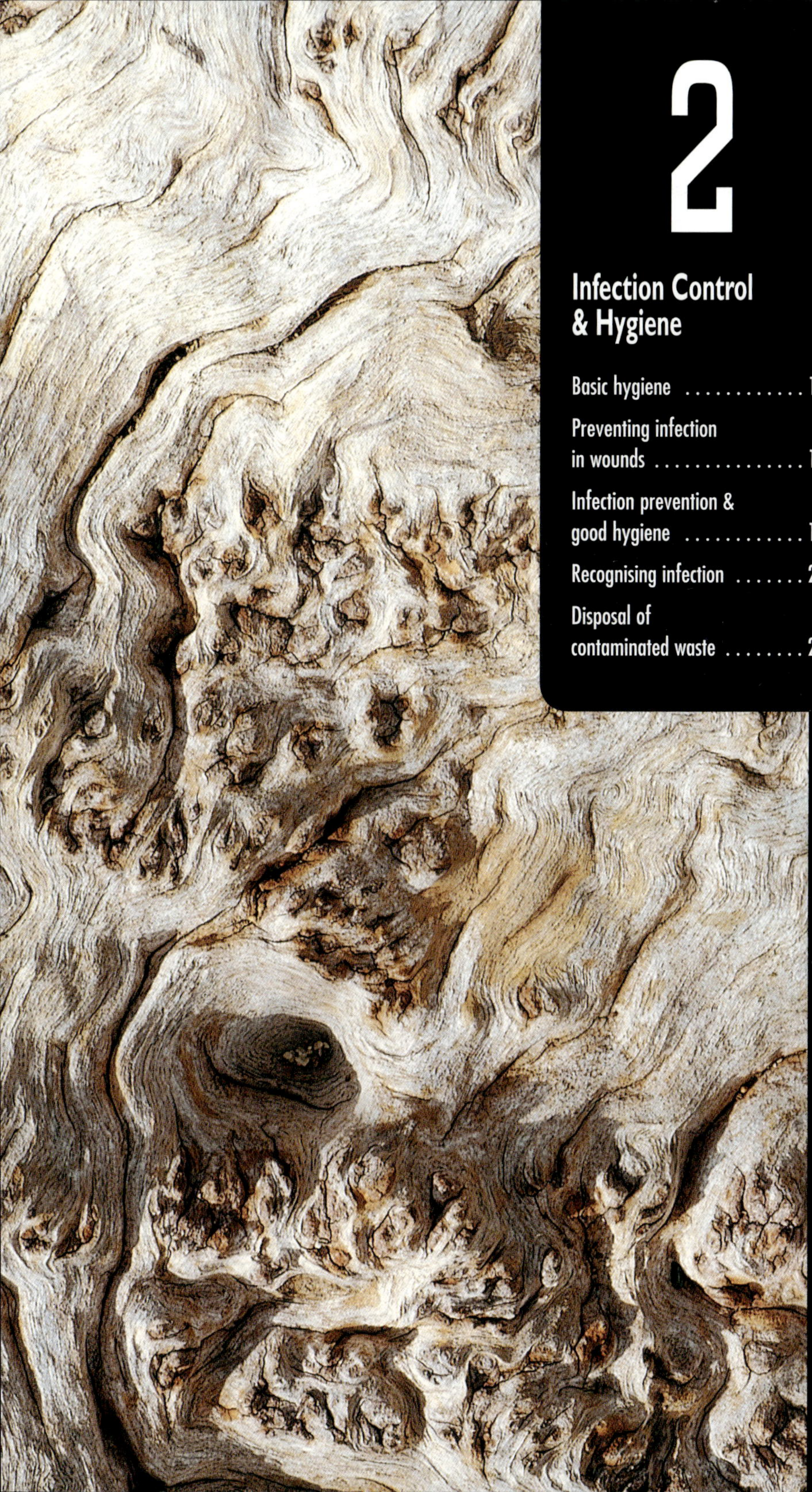

2

Infection Control & Hygiene

Preventing the spread of infection is very important—and even more so in remote areas. Contact with body fluids is quite common during first aid procedures. In urban areas, it is relatively easy to wash your hands carefully before and after first aid, and gloves may be readily available. In remote areas you may find that you have used all your gloves on the first day. Hand washing facilities may be difficult to set up and quite primitive. How will you manage?

Any body fluids (with the exception of sweat and tears) are potentially infectious and must be treated as such. Blood may contain viruses such as hepatitis and HIV. These may present a long-term problem for anyone who comes into contact with them. Blood may be present in other body fluids, even if only in minute quantities. Other body fluids, such as saliva, mucus, and faeces, may spread illnesses such as colds, flu, diarrhoea and vomiting. These conditions are more easily spread than blood-borne diseases, so contact with these fluids presents a more immediate problem. If you work to prevent the immediate problems, you will almost certainly prevent the long-term problems.

Basic hygiene

Hygiene is a basic habit of life for most of us; however, in remote areas it takes on a new significance. Without hot and cold running water, hygiene takes more effort and must be well planned to be effective.

Hygiene in remote areas can be divided into basic categories:

- personal hygiene
- camp craft
- first aid hygiene

Hygiene can be simply described as the techniques used to ensure that people living and working closely together, do not **all** become ill when one of them is sick.

The major rule of hygiene is WASH YOUR HANDS. The aim is to stop the spread of germs and to stop body fluids transferring from one person's body to another. Hand washing in a camp setting can be fairly difficult to set up, and even more difficult to enforce. A basin with water and disinfectant and nailbrush placed near the toilet area is an effective way to start.

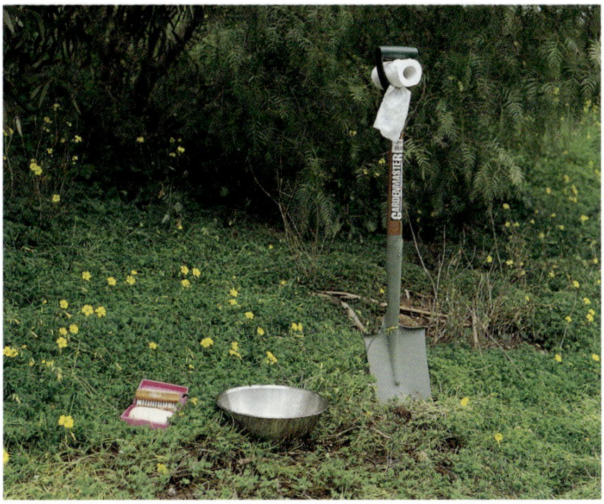

Another basic rule is not to share utensils, including water bottles. Now that water bladders are commonplace, it is easier to drink out of the container without contaminating it. However, it may be better to ensure that everyone drinks out of their own mug, not the common container. Try to segregate one water bottle/utensil for collecting water to reduce water contamination.

Additionally, when using untreated water, consider the possibility of hepatitis A infection. Hepatitis A is a disease that affects the liver and occurs when the virus is taken in by mouth.

It can be spread when people with the virus don't wash their hands thoroughly after going to the toilet, eat non-cooked food contaminated by an infectious person, eat shellfish from contaminated waters or drink contaminated water.

If a water supply comes from an untreated source, such as a lake or river, it may be contaminated by human faeces. Always boil water, or use purification tablets or a water purifier before drinking.

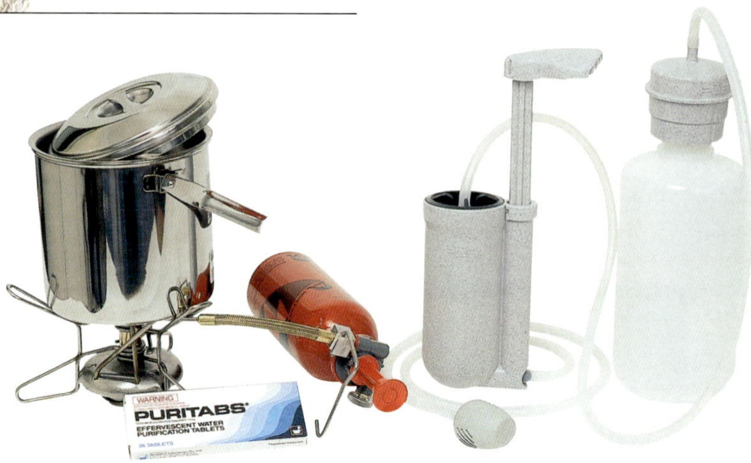

One very important aspect of hygiene is to try to wash your body each day. Fungal infections and chafing do not seem to affect a clean body as much as they do one that is rarely washed. It can be a very simple matter to wash and dry your face, underarms, genital area and feet when you get dressed in the morning. It takes less than 100 ml of water and only a couple of minutes, but can save days of pain and discomfort.

Preventing infection in wounds

In remote areas the way in which wounds are managed may mean the difference between the wound becoming infected or not.

A basic knowledge of wound care can assist in the prevention of infection and optimise recovery. Any wound must be thoroughly cleaned as soon as possible using clear fresh water or saline if you have it.

In hot, moist conditions such as tropical areas, wounds may easily become infected and therefore require redressing more frequently than, for example, in alpine areas.

Minor wounds such as a scratch from a twig or a small cut can be dealt with effectively provided basic hygiene and commonsense wound care is followed. Antiseptic preparations, such as povidone-iodine, may be used to assist in the prevention of infection particularly if your venture into a remote area is prolonged.

Major wounds such as deep and/or very dirty wounds will need to be cleaned as thoroughly as possible, have antiseptic applied and be covered. However, if bleeding is severe, the priority must be to stop the bleeding. Deep and/or very dirty wounds occurring in remote areas should be covered but not closed, as the risk of infection is very high—some of the most serious infections (e.g. tetanus and gas gangrene) thrive in a dark, moist, low-oxygen environment. Medical attention should be arranged as soon as possible *(see p. 150—managing wounds).*

The body is usually able to destroy minor accumulations of germs in a wound but not if there are solid particles of dirt remaining in the wound. Infected wounds must be referred to medical aid.

Infection can occur in the wound about six hours after the incident, when germs that have contaminated the wound begin to multiply and invade surrounding tissue.

Infection prevention and good hygiene during prolonged care

Providing prolonged care for casualties requires a lot of thought and preparation to prevent infection—for you, the casualty or any other member of the group. There will be many issues to consider. These include:

- **toiletting**—faeces is a potentially infectious substance and must be treated with care—wear gloves, if possible, and wash your hands
  - is the casualty capable of helping him/herself?
  - is there a family member or close friend who may be willing to help?
- **body washing**—the casualty will need the opportunity to have a wash each day; it will boost their morale, and help stop infections, chafing and 'nappy rash'
- **oral hygiene**—ensure that the casualty's teeth are cleaned regularly; if they are unconscious, you will need to wipe mouth and gums with a damp cloth at least once a day—maybe more frequently if mouth is very dry

- **menstruation**—if female casualty is unconscious you will need to check on this; if possible checks should be carried out by another female
- **contact lenses**—if the casualty wears these, you may need to assist with removal and cleaning; always ensure you have washed your hands first; if casualty unconscious:
  - check their eyes carefully
  - eyes must be kept moist and shut
  - you may need to remove contact lenses—only do this if you know how

  Note: Your local optometrist may be able to give you a lesson. If in doubt, do you have the means to call for advice?
- **pressure area care** (wound prevention)—any area of the body that is subjected to prolonged pressure will break down; this raw area needs to be treated like any other wound—cleaned and dressed at least daily; turning casualty from side to side every couple of hours will help prevent this problem; keeping the body clean and dry will also help

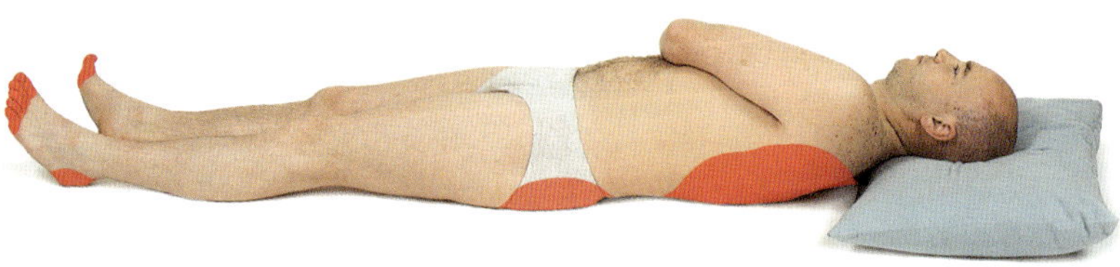

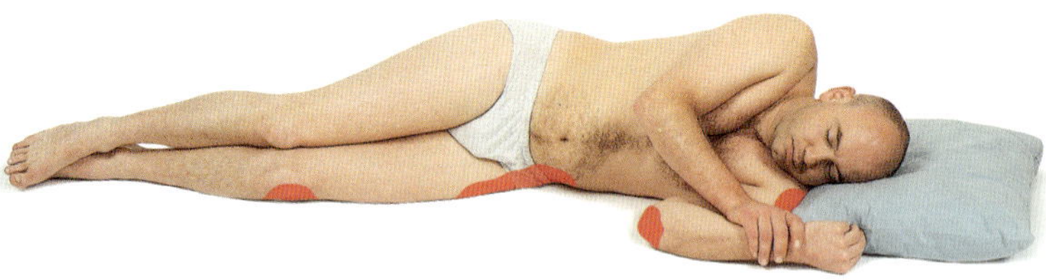

- **food and fluid intake**—ensure casualty drinks plenty of fluids; think carefully about what food you offer them with the aim to prevent further problems such as constipation; if anyone in the group has an upset stomach, diarrhoea or vomiting, be scrupulous about keeping utensils separate and washing up very carefully

Recognising infection

Wound infections can present major problems in remote areas. It is preferable to prevent them occurring. However, if infection has occurred, try to recognise it early and treat it before it becomes serious. Signs and symptoms of infection include:

- pain—progressively getting worse and often described as throbbing
- swelling around wound
- redness around wound—if redness appears to form streaks up the limb, infection is becoming quite serious
- heat around wound—skin feels much hotter than skin on other parts of body
- fever—if this develops, infection has spread to rest of body—this is serious

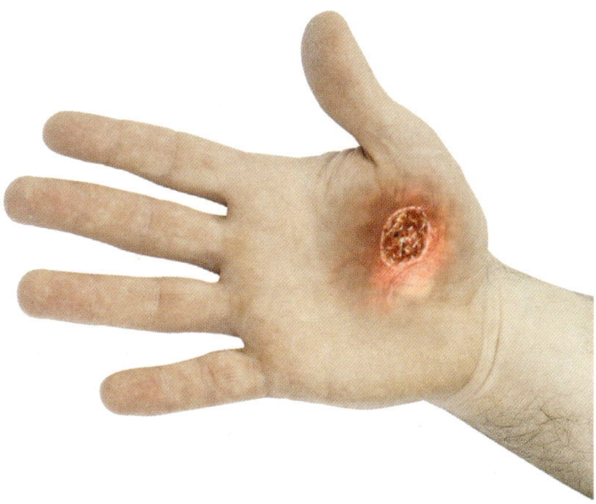

If any of these signs and symptoms occur, wound cleaning and dressing should be carried out more carefully and frequently—as often as 4 times a day may be necessary. Medical opinion must be sought as soon as possible. Great care must be taken to ensure that the infection is not spread to other members of the party—the first aider is most at risk.

Disposal of contaminated waste

Any waste must be bagged in plastic, carried out and placed in a rubbish bin. If the waste is heavily contaminated it should be double bagged. Any contaminated sharp objects need special care to ensure that no-one else is injured and potentially infected. Place the object in a puncture-proof container—e.g. empty drink bottle that is large enough to fully enclose it. It can then be bagged with the rubbish.

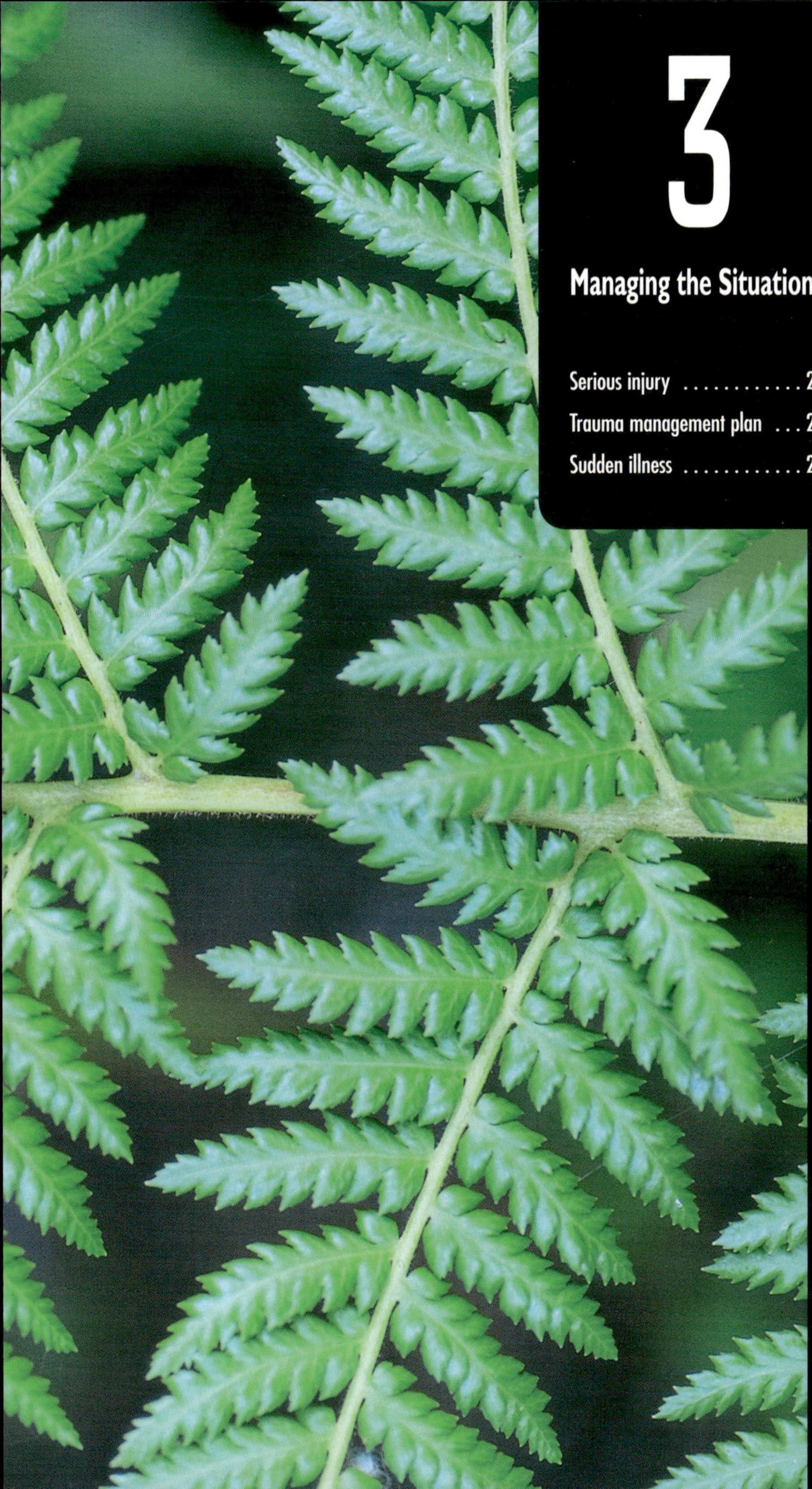

3

Managing the Situation

Having to manage a situation where a member of your party has suffered serious injury or become severely ill, in an environment where help is many hours away, is a daunting prospect.

A situation like this—compounded by bad weather, limited resources or the inability to communicate immediately with emergency organisations—can turn an exciting and pleasant outdoor activity into a frightening and overwhelming experience. While there is no magical formula or set of rules governing every situation, there are principles and actions we can apply that may help to stabilise the situation. In a case when a person has been seriously injured or has become suddenly severely ill, these principles and actions may contribute to saving their life.

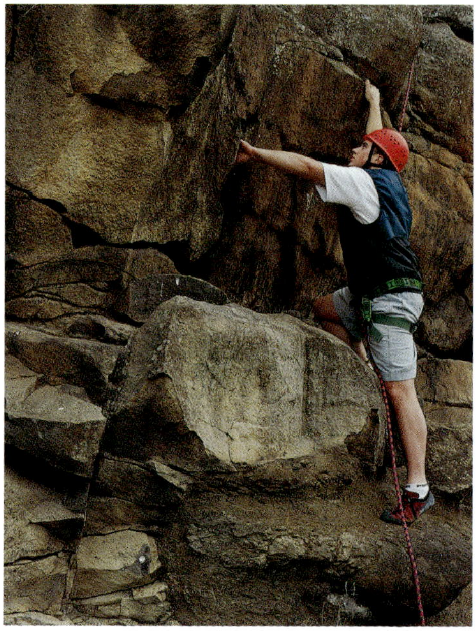

In this chapter we will consider managing the situation in which a member of a party has been seriously injured or has suddenly become ill.

Serious injury

How does one identify serious injury? The answer is essentially to believe the evidence before your eyes. If the casualty is unconscious, blood is pouring out of them, they are breathing with difficulty or limbs are apparently broken, they are seriously injured. When medical help is not readily available the problem is intensified. In this situation we need to identify the problem and initiate the appropriate management.

Before deciding on the management required for the seriously injured casualty we need to consider the following:

1 If there was enough force to cause the injury, it may also have caused other more serious and potentially life-threatening injuries.

2 Wherever possible do not move the seriously injured casualty. Not all injuries are apparent and the consequences of movement to the casualty with serious injuries may be disastrous. If you are able, and it is safe to do so, manage them where they are. There may be times when the casualty cannot be managed in the position or location found, but movement of a seriously injured casualty should not be undertaken lightly.

3 In a situation where someone is seriously injured and there are a limited number of people to assist, the priority must be to control life-threatening conditions such as bleeding. Once that is achieved or if there are sufficient numbers in the party, emergency services should be contacted immediately.

   There is a limit to what can be achieved for a seriously injured person in the field. Their survival may depend on the speedy application of skilled first aid, the provision of medical aid at the site by emergency services and transport to hospital with minimum delay.

4 Use all available resources to manage the situation. In some situations the first aid material carried by the party may, by necessity, be limited and the party will need to improvise using material at hand—towels, t-shirts or similar can be used as pads to stop bleeding; packs, sleeping bags and mats can be used to support broken bones in the position found; waist and shoulder straps from packs can be used in place of bandages to immobilise broken limbs.

In a situation where the casualty has multiple injuries the combined efforts of every member of the party may be needed to manage the problems.

The above points underpin a planned and organised approach that may be referred to as a trauma management plan. A trauma management plan is designed to ensure that the most serious or life-threatening problems are quickly identified and treated and that the casualty is examined from head to toe for injuries that are not readily apparent. Injuries will then be treated in order of seriousness.

Trauma management plan

Assess the situation

In looking at what happened—for example, a fall of approximately five metres—is it reasonable to expect the casualty will be seriously injured? Can you see from where you are that the casualty is seriously injured—for example, is blood pouring out of several injuries? If the answer is yes, direct that emergency services be contacted. The assistance of the emergency services is required as soon as possible.

Believe the evidence before your eyes—if you believe that the injuries are serious, do not hesitate to begin to get help as soon as the situation allows. Any delay in calling for help will delay its arrival and possibly affect the casualty's chance of survival.

Check for any danger

In the rush to assist the casualty it is easy for danger to be overlooked. Those going to the aid of the casualty need to quickly check the scene for any danger to themselves. Certainly in the situation where someone is seriously injured, time is of the essence but rushing in without considering the risk to yourself and other rescuers may result in the situation becoming more desperate, if a rescuer is also injured.

Check that casualty can breathe effectively

If the casualty is conscious ask them 'Can you breathe all right?' If the answer is yes, ask them to take a deep breath.

If the casualty cannot breathe effectively the chest needs to be exposed and checked for injury. A severely injured casualty with a chest injury who cannot breathe effectively, is breathless, can only breathe with some effort, or whose breathing is hardly sufficient to cause the chest to rise, is best managed by carefully rolling them on to their injured side. If the casualty is unconscious they should be rolled onto their side to maintain a clear and open airway.

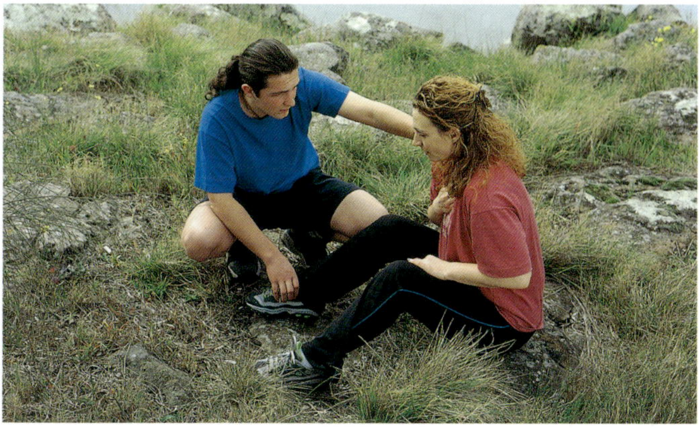

Stop bleeding

In remote areas a casualty who is bleeding heavily is at risk. The bleeding must be stopped quickly. Shirts and towels, for example, make effective pads to stop bleeding when held firmly on a wound.

Stabilise head and neck

An injury to the neck should be suspected:

- when the unconscious casualty has a head injury
- when any casualty has a serious head injury
- in all velocity accidents—that is, when force has been involved, such as in falls

While the absolute priority is to manage life-threatening problems such as inability to breathe effectively and/or severe bleeding, the possibility of a neck injury must be considered and the casualty's neck stabilised as soon as possible. This can be achieved quickly and effectively by holding the casualty's head steady with your hands. Material can also be placed alongside the head to help maintain position.

Improvised neck collars when applied by skilled, experienced operators can be of some value while the casualty is awaiting transport. However, unless the operators are well skilled and practised, the potential dangers of trying to apply a collar to a casualty who is suspected of having a neck injury outweigh the benefits. Stabilise the casualty's head by using your hands or packing to maintain the position of the head and stop movement.

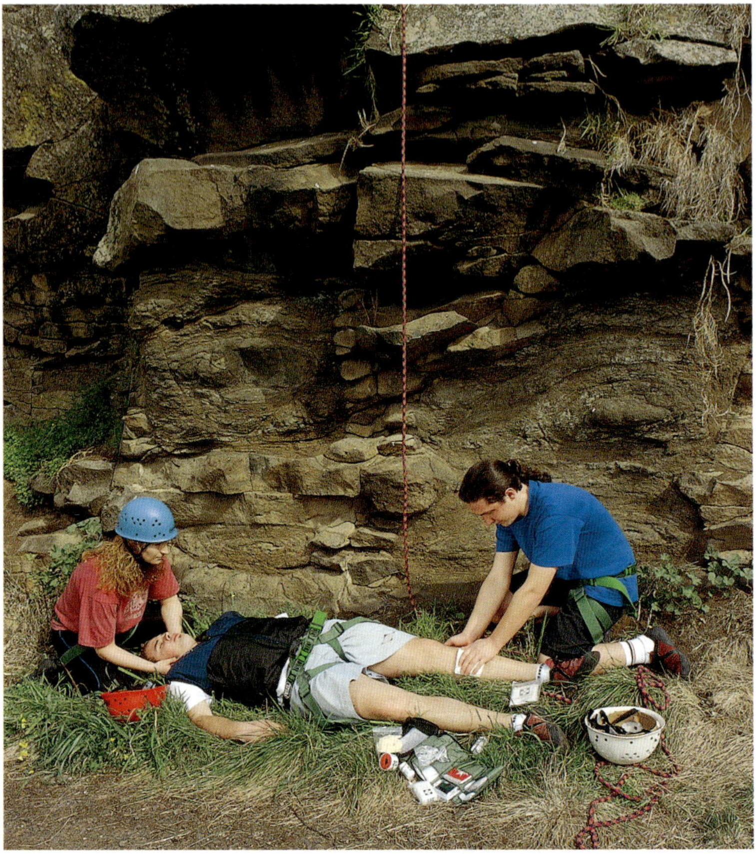

Check casualty for other injuries

As stated previously, if there has been enough force to cause obvious injuries it is quite possible that the casualty has sustained other injuries that are not readily apparent. It is important to quickly and thoroughly check the casualty from head to toe for other serious injuries.

Small wounds that are not bleeding are not a matter of priority and should not interfere with the process. Similarly, suspected broken bones which are identified can be managed later.

The priority is to make sure that there are no other heavily bleeding wounds.

History

Much is made of obtaining a history from the casualty concerning allergies, existing medical conditions, medications and so on. While this may be of value at a later time it is not a priority when managing a seriously injured casualty. The aim is to keep them alive. The first aider must direct all their attention and skill to managing the injuries.

Once the first aider has managed all injuries and the casualty is protected, attention can then be given to collecting a medical history. As the immediate dangers have in part been addressed by the first aider, the ambulance service and hospital staff will be able to devote time to gaining further information about the casualty's medical history.

Sudden illness

When a member of a party becomes suddenly ill, the first aider needs to identify the problem, determine the severity, and formulate a management strategy. It must be emphasised that identifying the problem does not mean diagnosing the condition. For example, where a member of the party develops chest pain, the problem is chest pain. The chest pain could be caused by indigestion, back injury, muscle strain, heart attack, collapsed lung, or a ruptured oesophagus. What is causing the pain is often difficult and time consuming even for physicians in a hospital to determine. For the first aider in the field it is neither reasonable nor realistic to expect to be able to 'diagnose' what is causing the pain.

Determining the severity of an illness and the threat it poses to the casualty is not an easy process.

While first aiders are often concerned about over-responding and calling for help when the casualty's condition may subsequently be diagnosed by a doctor as not life-threatening, the consequences of underestimating the problem could be disastrous.

In assessing the individual who has suddenly become ill the first aider needs to:

1 Believe the evidence before your eyes. We may not know what is making the person sick, but if they look sick, then they are sick.

2 Ask them how they feel. Ask them where they would place themselves on a scale of 1–10 where 10 is the worst they could feel. If they place themselves at 7 or 8 they feel very sick.

3 Ask have they ever felt like this before. If the response is yes, ask what caused it. It would be reasonable to be alarmed if they told you, for example, that they feel the same as when they had a kidney infection. If the response is 'No, I have never felt like this before', ask what they think is wrong. If they think they may be having a heart attack, take appropriate action.

4 Ask if they have any pain. If the answer is yes, again the scale of 1–10 can be used to determine the severity. Pain is a clear indicator that something is wrong. While constant, mild pain can be debilitating over a period of time, severe pain can weaken a casualty quickly. Pain relief is, in many cases, difficult to achieve in the field.

5 Do they have a fever, or feel hot? If you don't have a thermometer use the back of your hand to determine if they are hot. In a remote area, a casualty with an elevated temperature is a serious problem.

6 Can they breathe without difficulty, or do they have pain on taking a deep breath? If the casualty's ability to breathe is in any way impaired they must be viewed as seriously ill.

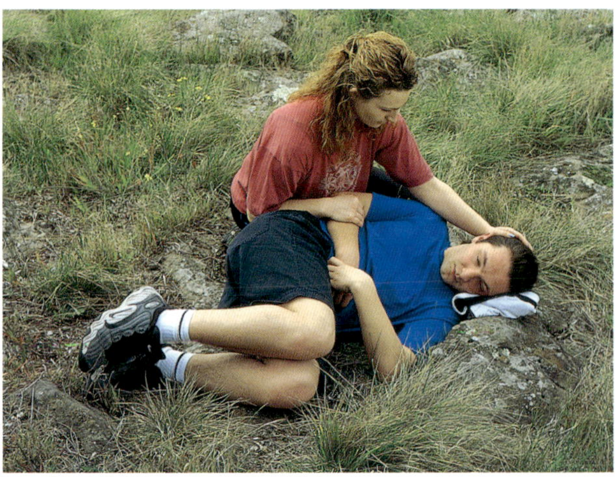

The decision to abort the activity and begin the process of contacting help to organise an evacuation should be promptly made with a casualty who:

- has a reduced level of consciousness
- cannot breathe properly
- has chest pain/discomfort
- is in severe pain
- has frequent vomiting or diarrhoea
- has a fever/chills
- is unable to walk

The decision of whether to obtain help is more difficult if the casualty feels unwell and has some difficulty keeping up with the group, but has none of the features listed above.

The fact that a casualty is ill must be recognised. To continue the activity may cause the casualty's condition to worsen or expose them to risk through an inability to concentrate on what they are doing.

In situations like this, when the decision is not clear and there is no obvious serious problem, it is best to stop, allow the casualty to rest, and reassess the situation after, say, four hours rest.

If after resting the casualty feels no better or feels worse, the decision to stop the activity and get the casualty out of the field becomes the priority.

In managing the casualty while awaiting the arrival of emergency services, there are some general actions that need to be taken. They include:

- protecting the casualty from the environment—heat, cold and wind
- ensuring the casualty is comfortable
- ensuring the provision of fluids, if appropriate, and toilet facilities
- providing ongoing reassurance

The person who becomes ill in a situation where medical care is not readily available is dependent for their care and safety on the other members of the party. In this situation the first aider needs to recognise their own limitations. To expect to be able to diagnose the casualty's condition is not realistic. Believe your eyes: 'if they look sick, they are sick'. If they are sick to the point that the casualty and the first aider are concerned, consider getting help. Initiate appropriate first aid management for the problem, protect the casualty from further injury and the environment, maintain their comfort and provide reassurance until help arrives.

By concentrating on issues that have a direct effect on the casualty the first aider can achieve a great deal.

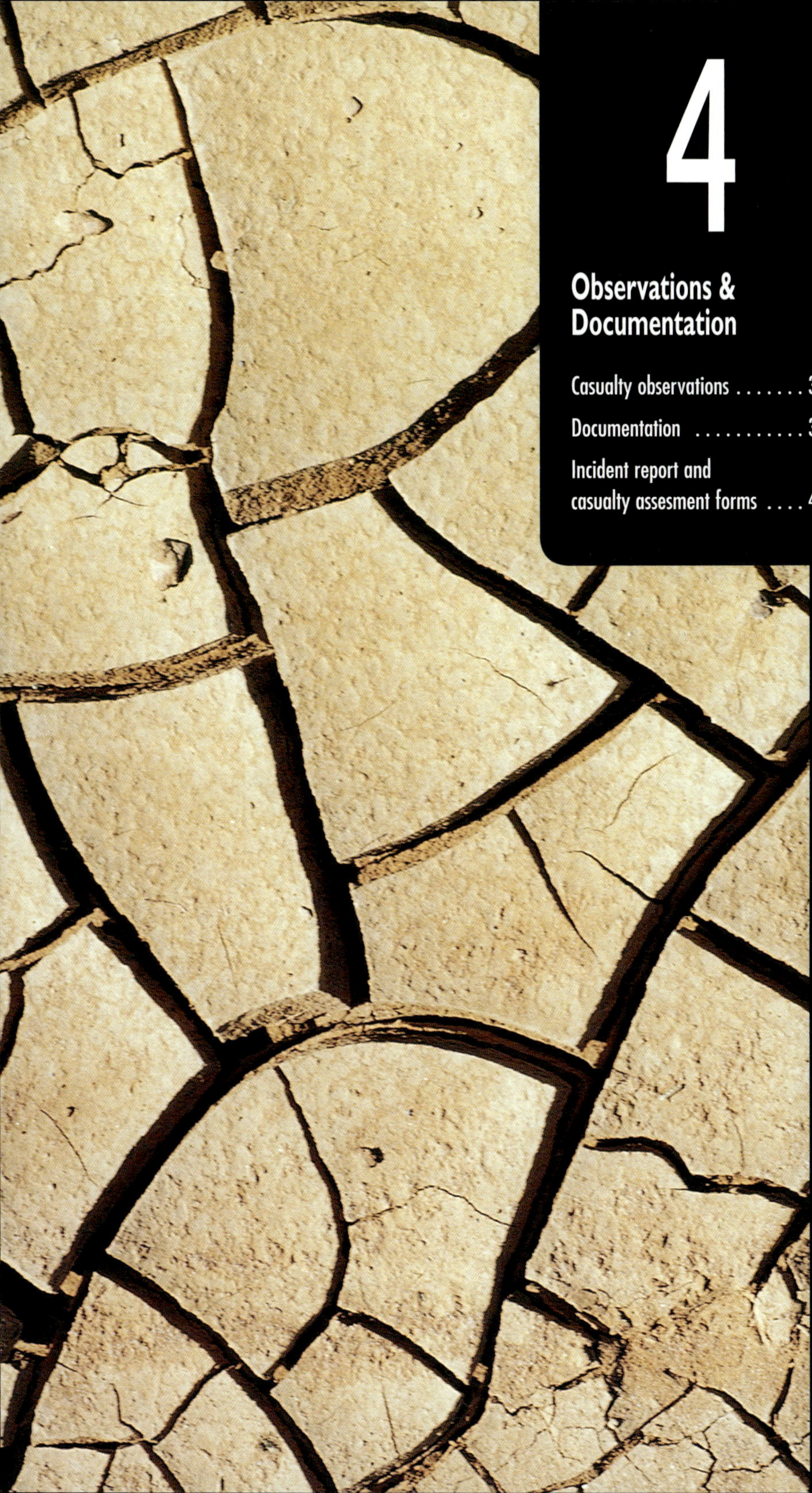

4

Observations & Documentation

In any situation in which a person has been injured or becomes seriously ill, the first aider's principal concerns are to:

- keep the casualty alive
- contact emergency services
- protect the casualty from the prevailing weather
- keep the casualty as comfortable as possible

To achieve this, the first aider will need many skills and abilities.

Always remember:

- keep your first aid training current
- do not go beyond your first aid training
- obtain the casualty's consent before administering first aid
- if consent for treatment is refused by the casualty and the situation is serious, you should call for help and gain advice from a health care professional
- document all management given and, in the case of a fatality, document all the circumstances

Note: It is the right of any person to refuse treatment. However, if the casualty is a minor, consent is assumed, especially if you are in loco parentis (e.g. a teacher in charge of students).

Casualty observations

Initial first aid management, prior to the arrival of emergency services, will be based on the first aider's initial observations of the casualty and the overall situation.

Once initial observations are recorded, the frequency of further observations will depend on the casualty's condition and the duration of care required. It is suggested that, initially, 15 minute observations are taken. However, if the casualty's condition is serious, more important tasks may take precedence.

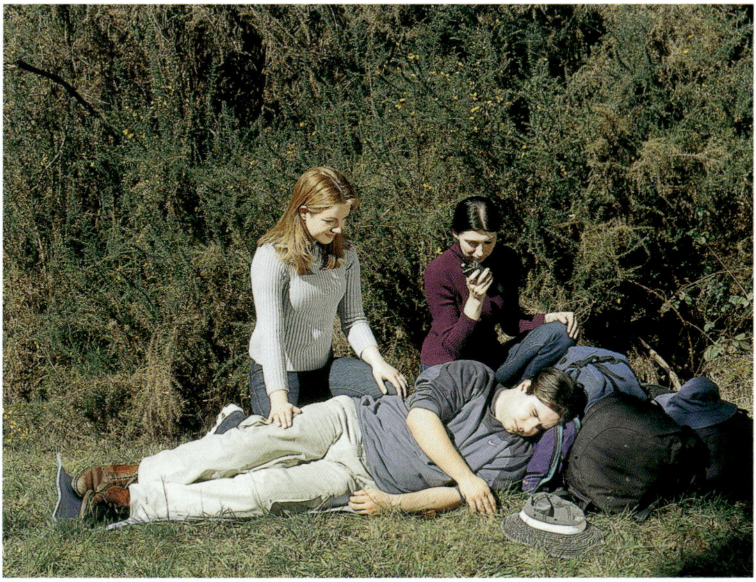

Never be afraid to ask for help or advice. If you have any form of communication equipment with you, it may be appropriate to call the local doctor, pharmacist, hospital, or Royal Flying Doctor Service (RFDS) for advice. If you have called for emergency rescue services, do not hesitate to continue to communicate with them—they will almost certainly want to be advised of any change in the casualty's condition or the condition of the rest of the party.

Important observations for the first aider to record include:

1 Is the casualty conscious or unconscious?

- if the casualty is talking, they are conscious
- if their eyes open when you speak to them or gently shake them, they are conscious
- if they do not respond, they are unconscious and need first aid quickly.

2 Is the casualty breathing all right?

- if the casualty can speak several sentences without becoming breathless, they can breathe all right
- if the casualty is conscious but quiet ask them:

- 'can you breathe all right?'
- 'take a big breath'

- if they answer 'yes' and can take a big breath, they can breathe all right
- if the casualty cannot breathe properly, attempt to manage the problem, for example:
  - chest injury—manage the injury
  - consider posture, loosen tight clothing
  - asthma—reliever puffer medication (via a spacer if available)

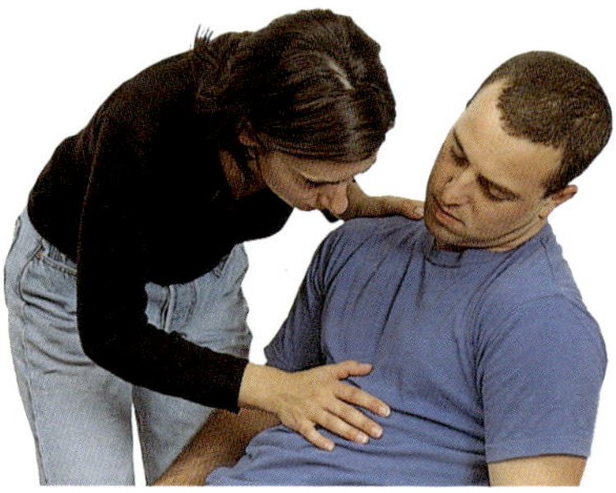

Observe breathing, count the number of breaths the casualty takes in one minute and record—breathing in and out counts as one breath. If this cannot be achieved, then observe and record the type of breathing—noisy, quiet, slow or fast.

3 How does the casualty look and feel?

- if you think the casualty looks sick then the casualty is sick:
  - does the casualty look apprehensive, frightened or excessively tired?
  - is the skin sweaty or dry, or hot to touch?
  - does the casualty say they feel sick—how sick?
  - does the casualty have any pain—if so where?

Other observations which may be recorded to assist in future management of the casualty are listed below.

Pulse

Count and record the casualty's pulse rate (beats per minute). If this cannot be achieved, then observe and record whether the pulse is weak, bounding, strong, regular or irregular.

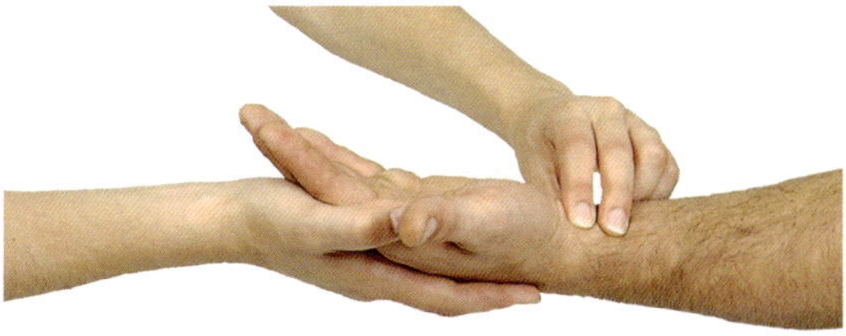

Pupils

If you are experienced in observing pupil size and reaction, check if the pupils react equally and quickly to light and if they are equal in size (some people may normally have unequal pupils); record observations.

Skin

Record the skin's appearance as:

- colour—pink, pale, blue, dusky, flushed, mottled, spotty
- condition—dry, clammy, sweaty
- temperature—hot, warm, cool or cold; if you are experienced in the use of thermometers and have one with you, take and record the temperature

Pain

Information documented about pain is often useful for ongoing management of the casualty. If possible ask the following questions:

1 Have you had the pain before—what did you do for it then?

2 Where is the pain?

3 Does it go anywhere else?

4 How long have you had it for?

5 How severe is the pain on a scale of 1–10, with 10 being the worst?

6 Does anything make it better or worse—position, heat or cold?

7 Describe the pain—sharp, throbbing, aching.

8 Do you have the pain all the time, or does it come and go?

9 Does the pain interfere with breathing or movement?

Fluid intake and output

If possible the volume of all fluid in and out of the body should be estimated and recorded. This includes drinks, urine, faeces, bleeding (including menstruation), vomit, even excessive sweating.

A description of the fluid should be included, such as appearance and amount. DO NOT attempt to measure faeces; simply estimate the amount—large, medium or small *(see p. 16)*. In a remote area, it is often helpful to note any type and amount of food eaten by the casualty.

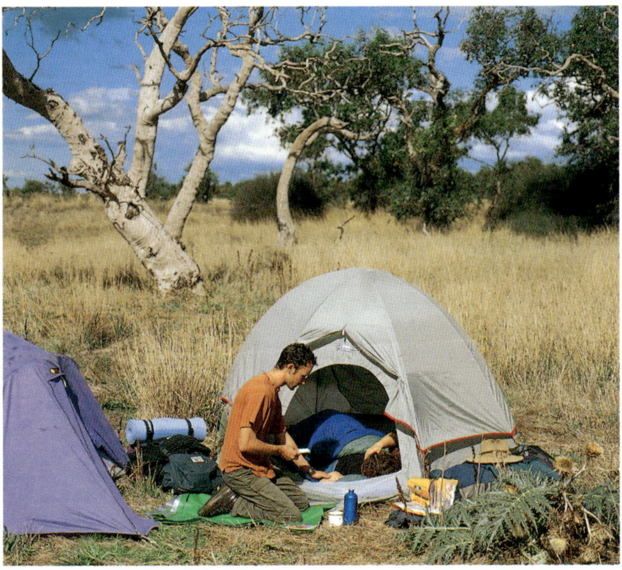

Documentation

Documenting the casualty's condition as soon as practicable after the incident will give medical aid a guide in establishing whether the condition is getting better or worse.

A record of the event written in plain language should be started as soon as possible after it is noticed the casualty is seriously ill or injured.

When handing over care of the casualty to another person, it will be necessary to provide both verbal and written information.

The written documentation should:

1 State casualty's name and age.

2 State time and date of incident.

3 State name of first aider.

4 Describe what occurred.

5 If possible, state location of incident.

6 Describe observations, for example:
   - difficulty breathing
   - appeared to be in pain—clutching chest
   - looked pale and skin felt cool and sweaty
   - could only lie down.

7 Describe what casualty complained of, for example:
   - could not breathe
   - wanted to vomit but could not
   - was frightened
   - having a heart attack.

8 List any other signs and symptoms observed.

9 Describe what actions were taken, for example:
   - emergency services were contacted for advice—note time
   - casualty was made as comfortable as possible
   - casualty was given small sips of water when thirsty.

10 Describe ongoing actions and any changes in the casualty's condition, for example:
   - more advice sought—note time
   - casualty complaining of feeling very cold—note time
   - any medication taken by casualty *(see p. 127)*.

11 Detail intake and output of food and fluid *(see p. 38)*.

12 State current immunisation—tetanus (if relevant to casualty's condition).

13 Detail existing medical conditions and/or allergies.

This type of record can be useful in developing a clear picture of what actually happened and should whenever possible be maintained.

In remote areas, the first aider may advise a casualty to see a doctor but this may not be possible for some time because of the remoteness. There will be situations in which the first aider will be consulted about seemingly minor problems which may not warrant documentation—for instance, a member of your party complains of a headache, but does not require any treatment. The temptation is not to document; however it is worth keeping a diary, journal or other daily record in which to note these occurrences. Otherwise it can be easy to lose track of such problems, which could linger, worsen or return.

If the worst happens and the casualty dies, written documentation will help the coroner establish time and cause of death. If a court case arises following an incident, written documentation will help you to remember what you did, and when and why you did it. In serious or potentially serious situations, it may be advisable to make two copies of your notes—one for you and one to go with the casualty.

Incident report and casualty assessment forms

Examples are shown on the following pages of report forms which may be used as a guide for the collation of observations and documentation.

Incident Report

Full name of casualty: ....

Age: ....   Male/Female: ....

Date and time of incident: ....

Location: ....

Emergency services contacted: yes/no date and time: ....

Method of contact: ....

Description of what happened: ....

Injuries/problem identified: ....

First aid given: ....

Other actions taken to assist casualty: ....

Relevant medical history (include allergies and medication): ....

....

Signature: ....

Print name: ....   Date: ....

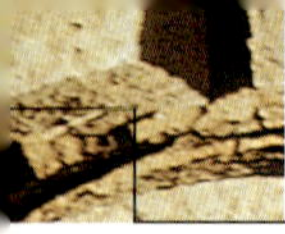

Observation Chart			
Time	Pulse: rate/rhythm/ strength	Respiration: rate/rhythm/ depth/noises	Skin: colour/temp./ condition

Observation Chart		
Intake: type/amount	Output: type/amount	Comments: pain/medication/ dressings/pressure area care/emotional state

Date .... Casualty's Name ....

Observation Chart							
	Time (15 minute intervals)	0	15	30	45	60	75
Eyes							
Observe for reaction while testing other reponses.	Open spontaneously						
	Open to speech						
	No response						
Movement							
	Obeys commands						
	No response						
Speech							
When testing responses, speak clearly and directly, close to the casualty's ear.	Responds sensibly to questions						
	Seems confused						
	Uses inappropriate words						
	Makes incomprehensible sounds						
	No response						
Pulse							
Take pulse at wrist on conscious casualty; at neck on unconscious casualty.	Beats per minute						
	Weak						
	Strong						
	Regular						
	Irregular						
Breathing							
Note rate and describe.	Breaths per minute						
	Quiet						
	Noisy						
	Easy						
	Difficult						

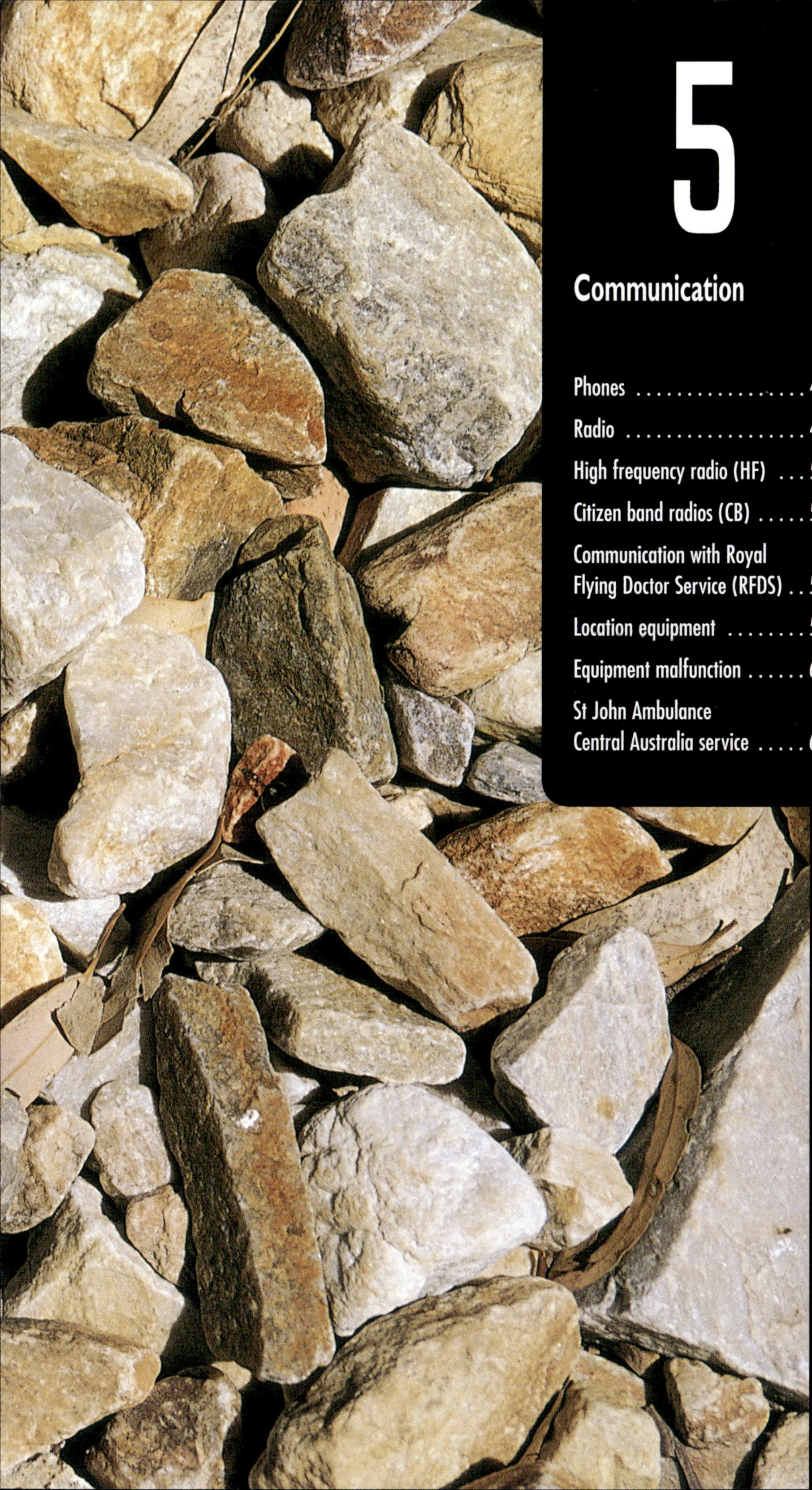

5

Communication

Communication methods used in remote areas can affect the welfare of a number of people—casualties, first aiders and other members of the group. Information communicated will usually fit into one of the following categories:

Danger—immediate, urgent, for the benefit of self, others and the casualty

Emergency medical assistance—help is required as soon as possible

Emergency medical advice—medical problem but not urgent enough for evacuation or medical attendance

Reassurance—possibly ongoing, for the benefit of self, others and the casualty

Monitoring—of casualty's condition over a period of time

It is essential when planning a trip that you choose the most appropriate communication equipment for the area where you are intending to travel. In addition you should have backup communication equipment for use in an emergency or for two-way communication if the group needs to split up.

There is a myriad of communication equipment that operates effectively, but only if correctly chosen for the environment in which you are to travel. This chapter provides you with information about various types of equipment that you may wish to consider for your proposed trip.

Note: Mobile phones, citizen band (CB) and ultra high frequency (UHF) radios have limited capabilities and should only be used as a backup to high frequency (HF) radio if you are planning to travel somewhere remote.

Phones

Mobile phone

When a group is travelling into a remote area, particularly without a vehicle, at least one mobile phone should be carried as a backup. Many popular areas of Australia, in particular south-eastern Australia, are mountainous or hilly—a mobile phone will almost always work from the top of the nearest high point from the top of the nearest high point (except where there are long distances between towns, e.g. Alice Springs and Tennant Creek). However, use of mobile phones is limited without power to recharge the battery.

Remember: Emergency services can be contacted from any functioning mobile phone by dialling 000.

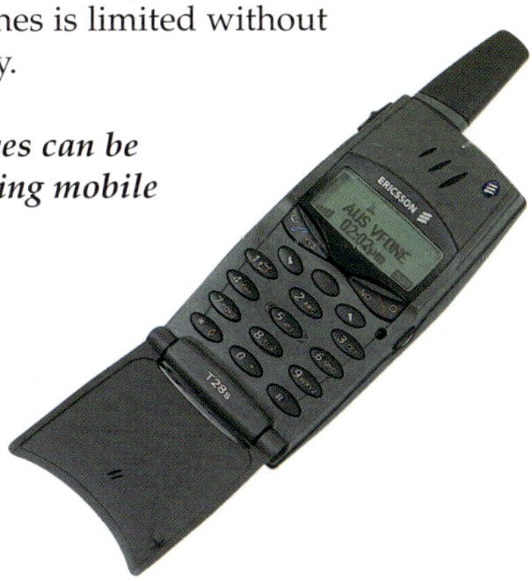

Satellite phone

The ability to communicate over long distances for an extended length of time requires spending a reasonable amount of money on good quality electronic equipment such as a satellite phone or HF radio set. A satellite phone has the advantage of being able to send and receive calls from almost anywhere at any time, whereas an HF set is restricted to working from a vehicle.

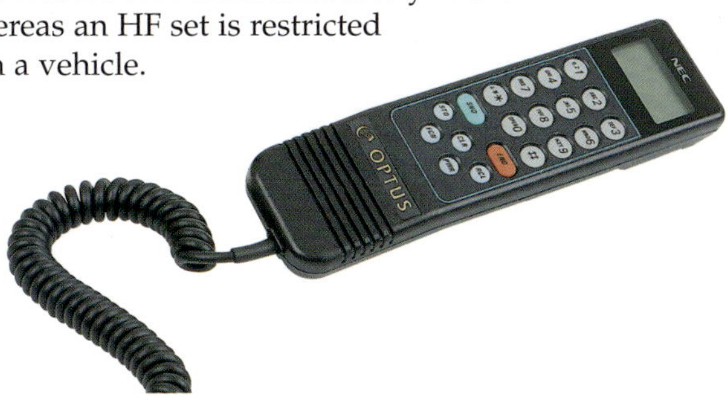

Radio

Radio frequency communications available for general use tend to fall into one of two categories: UHF (ultra high frequency) and HF (high frequency). Both have strengths and weaknesses.

Inclement weather conditions affect all radios. In particular:

- transmission should not be attempted during electrical storms
- external antenna systems and power supplies should be disconnected during electrical storms
- higher frequencies will usually be more successful at higher temperatures

Operating the radio

When calling for help by radio or telephone or when passing a message to another person, the content of your message is vital. It must be accurate and contain all details of the incident. This is extremely important in a remote area, as panic-induced messages or messages containing little information can delay emergency services. Distances in remote areas are far too great to take a chance that emergency services will assume any details that are missing from your message.

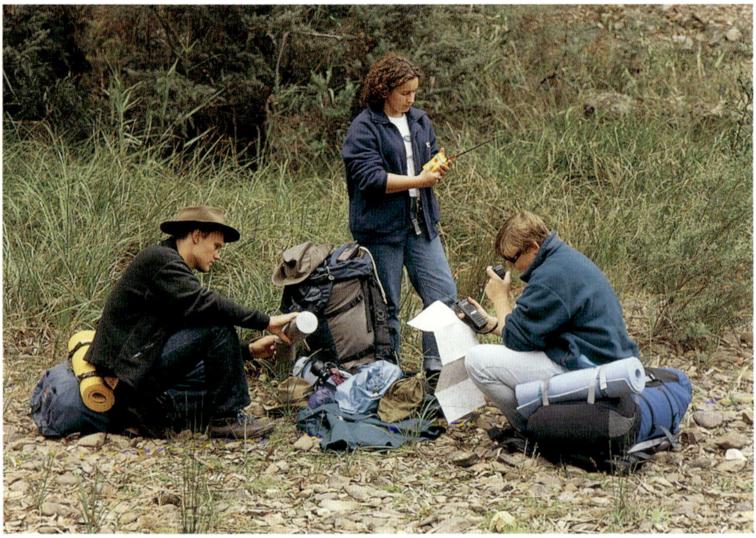

The key steps for transmitting a message are:

1. Think about, and if possible note down, what you will say.
2. Wait until no other stations are operating, unless your call is an emergency.
3. Press transmit button.
4. Speak the message clearly—keep the message as short as possible to conserve the battery life.
5. Release transmit button.
6. Listen for a reply.

It is important to keep to this order of using the radio—if you speak before pressing, the start of the message will be lost.

Alphabet

If you need to spell a word or communicate a group of letters over the radio, using the 'phonetic alphabet' will clarify the message. Any group of phonetics must be preceded by the pro-word 'I SPELL'.

A	Alpha	J	Juliet	S	Sierra
B	Bravo (BRAHvo)	K	Kilo (KEElo)	T	Tango
C	Charlie	L	Lima (LEEma)	U	Uniform
D	Delta	M	Mike	V	Victor
E	Echo	N	November	W	Whisky
F	Foxtrot	O	Oscar	X	X-ray
G	Golf	P	Papa (PaPA)	Y	Yankee
H	Hotel	Q	Quebec (KWIbeck)	Z	Zulu
I	India	R	Romeo		

Numerals

When pronunciation of numerals is required, the code word 'FIGURES' precedes the message. For giving the time it is preferred that the 24-hour clock is used.

For clarity in an emergency, use the following pronunciation of numerals (for numbers over 9 pronounce each numeral separately, e.g. 'WUN ZERO' instead of 'ten'):

0	ZE-RO	5	FIFE
1	WUN	6	SIX
2	TOO	7	SEV-en
3	TREE	8	AIT
4	FOW-er	9	NINE-er

Other hints for radio use

There is little need to use technical 'radio talk' but there are some standard, easily understood phrases and words:

OVER	my transmission is finished and I am listening
AFFIRMATIVE	yes
NEGATIVE	no
RECEIVED	your message was heard and understood
SAY AGAIN	please repeat the message
STAND BY	please wait and continue listening
OUT	finished transmission

High frequency radio (HF)

HF radios generally operate in the frequency range 2–30 MHz. Radio traffic can be effective over short or long distances, depending on the frequency, transmitter power, terrain, time of day, time of year, weather and solar activity. Frequencies from 2–6 MHz will usually cover most situations.

HF sets can incorporate many frequencies including those for the Royal Flying Doctor Service (RFDS) and other agencies' radiotelephone, outback/four wheel drive radio networks and many others. While not designed for the purpose, the sets can also be used for inter-vehicle communications but care should be taken not to interfere with other radio networks.

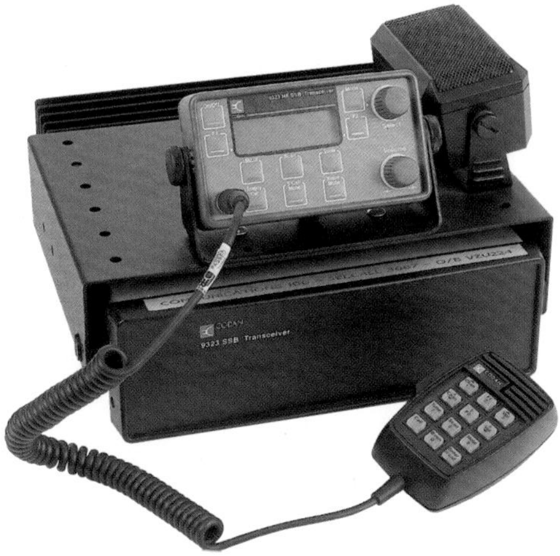

Some points to remember about HF radios:

- good for long-distance communications
- enhanced by clear atmospheric conditions
- impeded by electromagnetic forces, weather conditions, low voltage supply to the unit
- level of voice quality varies considerably (from good to very poor)
- antenna needs adjusting to suit each frequency
- restricted to vehicle-mounted unit
- frequencies very much subject to atmospheric conditions, but network control bodies have multiple frequencies to overcome this so communications can usually be achieved over hundreds of kilometres
- HF base stations at fixed locations are usually more powerful than vehicle-mounted radios so will generally have more difficulty receiving the weaker vehicle-mounted set

Citizens band (CB) radios

Citizen band radios are generally fitted to most buses, trucks and cars venturing into the outback. The radios are relatively cheap to buy and provide good intervehicle communication for short distances, up to 5–10 km in ideal circumstances.

Many farm and station properties also have CB radio facilities, especially UHF CB. CBs, however, are not generally suitable for urgent communications in a remote area because long distance coverage is particularly dependent on terrain and atmospheric conditions.

There are two types of CB radios, UHF and HF (AM/SSB).

UHF CB sets have a high quality voice signal, but are generally 'line of sight' dependent which essentially means you need to be within sight of the other party to establish communications.

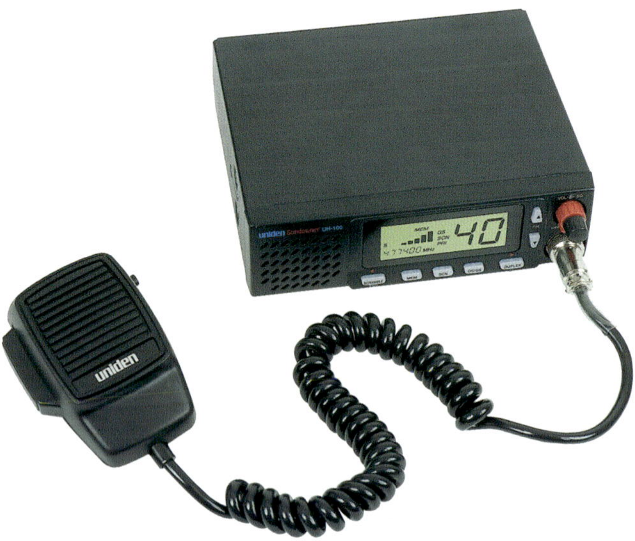

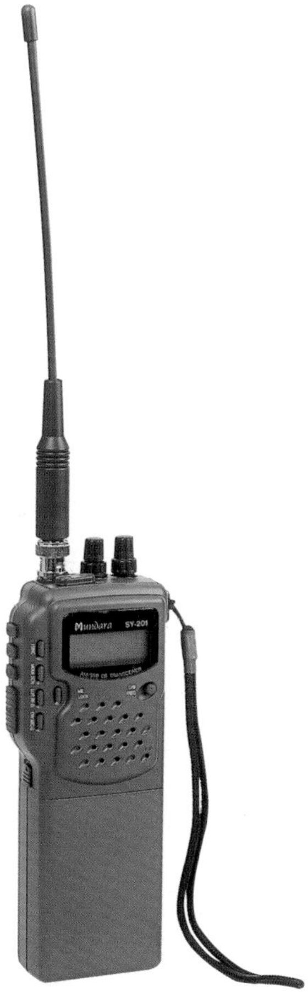

Some points to remember about UHF CB radios:

- line of sight communication only
- channel 5 is usually set aside for emergency transmission
- can be enhanced by use of a repeater network
- impeded by electromagnetic forces, electrical storms, densely particled atmospheres (such as smoke), buildings and mountains
- good level of voice clarity
- antenna tends to be pre-set to correct frequencies
- generally used for communicating over short distances

AM sets have the greatest chance of long distance transmissions, particularly if fitted with a 'side band' capability. Quality of transmission is variable with significant interference from overseas countries, especially in the outback desert areas.

Unfortunately because of the nature of its function, CB radio is often used for chatting. With spurious transmission being common, it can be difficult to get someone to take notice of an emergency transmission. Consequently it is not a reliable medium.

Communication with Royal Flying Doctor Service (RFDS)

Emergency communications via the Royal Flying Doctor Service (RFDS) can be made at any time. Calls of a non-urgent nature should only be made in office hours when there is staff to handle them.

Using HF radio to call RFDS:

1 Select the primary frequency of the station you wish to call and tune the antenna *(see p. 55)*.

2 In an emergency:

- use the Emergency Alarm Call Button on your radio—send the alarm for at least 20 seconds.

3 If within the operating hours of the station and the channel is clear of other conversations, you should be able to voice-call the station and get a reply.

4 A calling station may need to repeat emergency procedure at 3 minute intervals until RFDS base responds. The alarm alerts base station and other users of emergency call. Other users will stand down to allow call to proceed.

5 If no reply, keep trying other frequencies or stations.

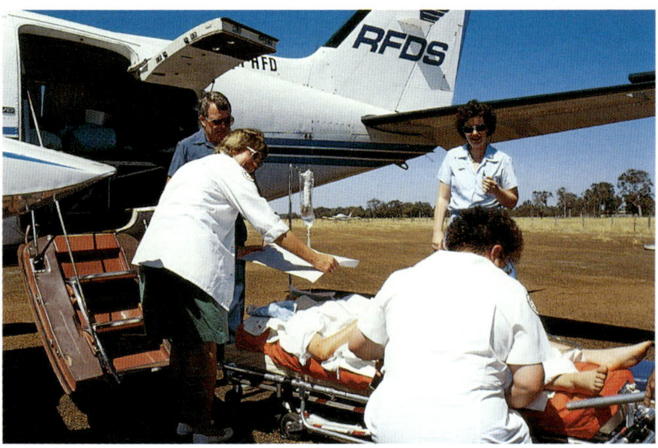

Frequencies

As RFDS frequencies are on high frequency radio, voices can sometimes become mixed in with radio static and other interference. When a message is being transmitted, it may be necessary at times to actually spell a word, a place name or the call sign of a calling station. The phonetic alphabet assists the user to understand a word more clearly *(see p. 49)*.

RFDS radio frequencies

	RFDS section	Primary frequencies daytime sign	Telephone number	Call
Cairns	Queensland	5145	07 4053 1952	VJN
Mt Isa	Queensland	5110	07 4743 2800	VJI
Charleville	Queensland	4980	07 4654 1233	VJJ
Broken Hill	NSW	4055	08 8080 1777	VJC
Alice Springs	Central	5410	08 8952 5355	VJD
Port Augusta	Central	4010	08 8642 2555	NVZ
Derby	Western	5300	1800 62 5800	VJB
Port Hedland	Western	5300	1800 625 8000	VKL
Carnarvon	Western	5360	Enq. 08 9414 6300	VJT
Meekatharra	Western	5360	08 9414 1300	VKJ
Kalgoorlie	Western	5360	08 9414 1300	VJQ

Frequencies and times of operation of Australian Outpost HF Radio Stations are subject to change without notice. When planning a trip, calling up the Internet web site www.pca.cc will provide you with up-to-date frequencies and current operating times of the stations.

If using the more expensive equipment, it is recommended that you study the manual and have some training on equipment. The various user networks generally require pre-registration and payment of a user fee, although there is no registration fee for the RFDS. Most have multiple frequencies allowing use at any time, but some are only staffed for limited hours. Don't forget that such equipment requires licensing annually with the Federal Government Australia Communications Authority.

Your message

Important points need to be included in your message when calling RFDS:

- date and time of message
- location of incident
- distance from a major town or landmark
- nature of emergency or difficulty
- number of casualties
- suspected nature and severity of injuries
- special hazards
- time of accident or incident if known
- primary and secondary casualty observations

The use of a message form may assist you in collecting and passing on important information to emergency services.

Message form

Describe location: ....

Name of district/area: ....

Distance from town or major landmark: .... km

north ☐ south ☐ east ☐ west ☐

of .... (describe town or landmark)

Incident/accident details: ....

Number of people injured: ....

Time of accident (if known): ....

Time this message written: ....

Notes about incident: ....

....

....

....

Message written by: ....

Once radio contact has been made to an RFDS base, the doctor will call the station.

When you speak with the doctor over the radio:

- have pen and paper ready
- have all the casualty's details ready
- be prepared to answer questions about casualty's condition
- listen carefully to doctor's instructions and write them down
- repeat doctor's instructions and ask any questions if unsure

Once the doctor has all relevant information he/she will either:

- arrange for you to manage the casualty using the RFDS medical chest and body chart located at most stations and/or,
- arrange to evacuate the casualty by air or other means

For information about how to use the RFDS medical chest and body chart *(see p. 128)*.

Location equipment

If all forms of verbal communication have been exhausted you will need to rely on equipment which could help rescuers locate you.

Location devices are used to attract the attention of anyone in range of hearing, seeing or electronic signals. Attention may be gained, for example, by blowing a whistle or using visual means, e.g. smoke, mirror or electronic communication equipment such as an Emergency Position Indicating Radio Beacon (EPIRB).

Emergency Position Indicating Radio Beacon (EPIRB)

The EPIRB is designed to help save your life if you get into trouble, by alerting rescue authorities and indicating your location using satellite detection. There are various types of EPIRB on the market that are designed for specific purposes. It is important that you choose the EPIRB that is best suited for your intended use and follow the instructions for use and for testing, battery replacement and registration regulations.

Because the EPIRB is not capable of transmitting speech, it should always be regarded as supplementary to, not a substitute for, radio or other reliable communication equipment. Once activated the EPIRB should not be turned off until location and rescue are complete.

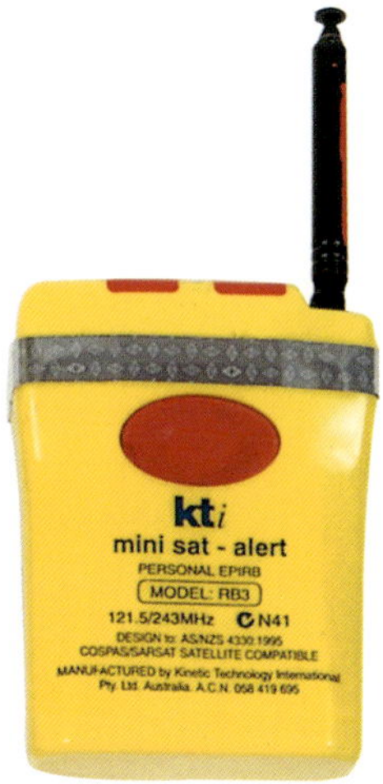

Whistle

Whistle blasts are effective when trying to attract the attention of others nearby. Every member of the group should carry a whistle at all times in case they become separated from the group. The international distress signal is three short blasts at regular intervals.

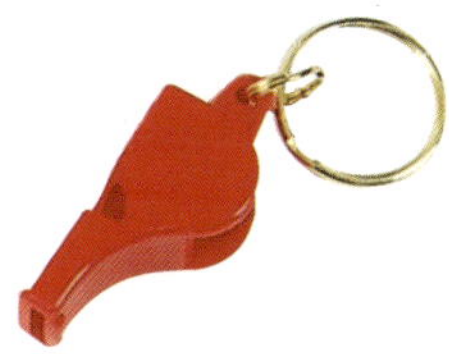

Reflective devices

Mirrors and/or any other reflective material may be useful for attracting attention as a last resort.

'V' Distress Sheet

A 'V' Distress Sheet is readily visible from the air and should be a rectangular fluorescent orange–red sheet of material with the letter 'V' in black. The letter 'V' should not be less than 760 mm high and the strokes forming the 'V' not less than 130 mm wide. The sheets should not be smaller than 1.8 x 0.5 m.

Although primarily intended to increase the chances of locating small craft from the air, the sheet may also be exhibited by any person or group in any manner that will best attract attention.

Smoke

Attracting attention with fire and/or smoke is regarded as a distress signal. Light three fires 30 metres apart in a triangle or in a line. Fires can be started by using fuel, oil, dead wood and grass. They can be used day or night in most places, even in snow country. The fire will be shown as a 'column of smoke' by day and a 'pillar of fire' by night.

Check with State/Territory Fire Authorities for current restrictions regarding lighting of fires. Take care—**do not** create a disaster with fire:

- **DO NOT** leave a fire unattended
- extinguish fire before leaving the site

Flares/lights

Flares are commercially available and it is advisable to purchase some prior to an extended trip. Improvised flares can be made by lighting kerosene soaked rags. Flares can be used to light an airstrip to allow emergency services aircraft to land safely. Full details of laying out an airstrip are explained in detail in chapter nine *(see p. 112)*.

Signal methods—ground-to-air/air-to-ground

If radio communication with the pilot of an aircraft is not possible, location aids such as emergency codes may be used. These codes are explained in detail in the chapter concerning preparation for rescue *(see p. 107)*.

Equipment malfunction

All electronic equipment of any size and expense requires careful installation and maintenance. The equipment should be protected from the elements (e.g. cold, heat, dust, salt), and care taken of the antenna and wiring. Such equipment is prone to malfunction and breakdown and it is wise to carry the equipment manual. For smaller devices spare parts are rarely required except for batteries.

For larger equipment such as a radio it may be appropriate to carry a spare or temporary antenna, power cabling and coaxial cable. The same piece of wire may act as a temporary antenna or a spare power cable depending on requirements.

Batteries used in portable equipment are likely to be the main problem. Careful warming of a battery may gain a few vital minutes of additional life.

For larger communication equipment the size, weight and expense are considerable. The most common problems for vehicle- mounted sets are broken or loose wiring or poor earthing. Attention to securing the mounting while installing will usually be rewarded with high reliability. Antenna size and dust are also common problems or the antenna may be physically damaged, e.g. by overhanging branches.

St John Ambulance Central Australia service

The St John Ambulance service in Central Australia provides Alice Springs, Tennant Creek and surrounding remote areas with routine and emergency road transport evacuations. To coordinate all road transport evacuations St John Ambulance service provides the region with a 24-hour communications network. This facility has been extended to the VJD call sign *(see p. 55)*, which is managed by the RFDS during normal working hours. All after hours, weekend and public holidays are managed by St John Ambulance Alice Springs, on behalf of RFDS.

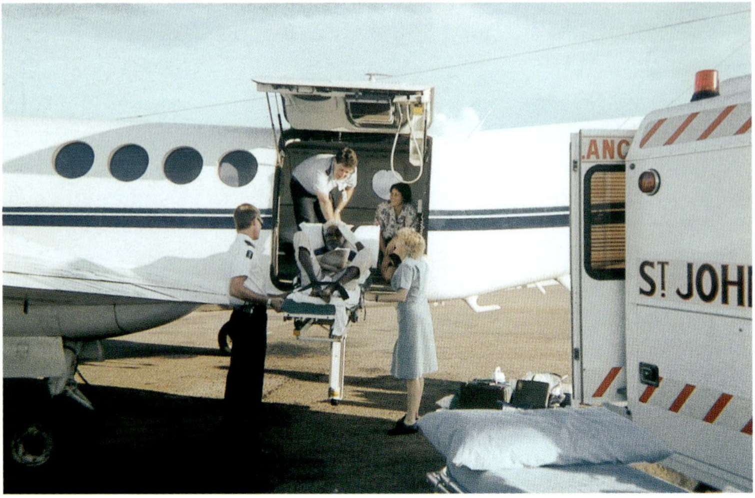

In recent years HF radio has been supplemented in many areas by satellite telephone systems. However the communications centre still maintains an HF system to provide coverage in remote communities and to the travelling public.

The after hours communications provided by St John Ambulance also enable coordination of medical consultations from remote areas to the District Medical Officers. It may be appropriate, as a result of the consultation, that the casualty is evacuated by road or the RFDS to the nearest major medical facility or the nearest interstate capital city. Either type of evacuation would be organised and coordinated by the St John Ambulance Communications Officer.

6

Safety & Survival

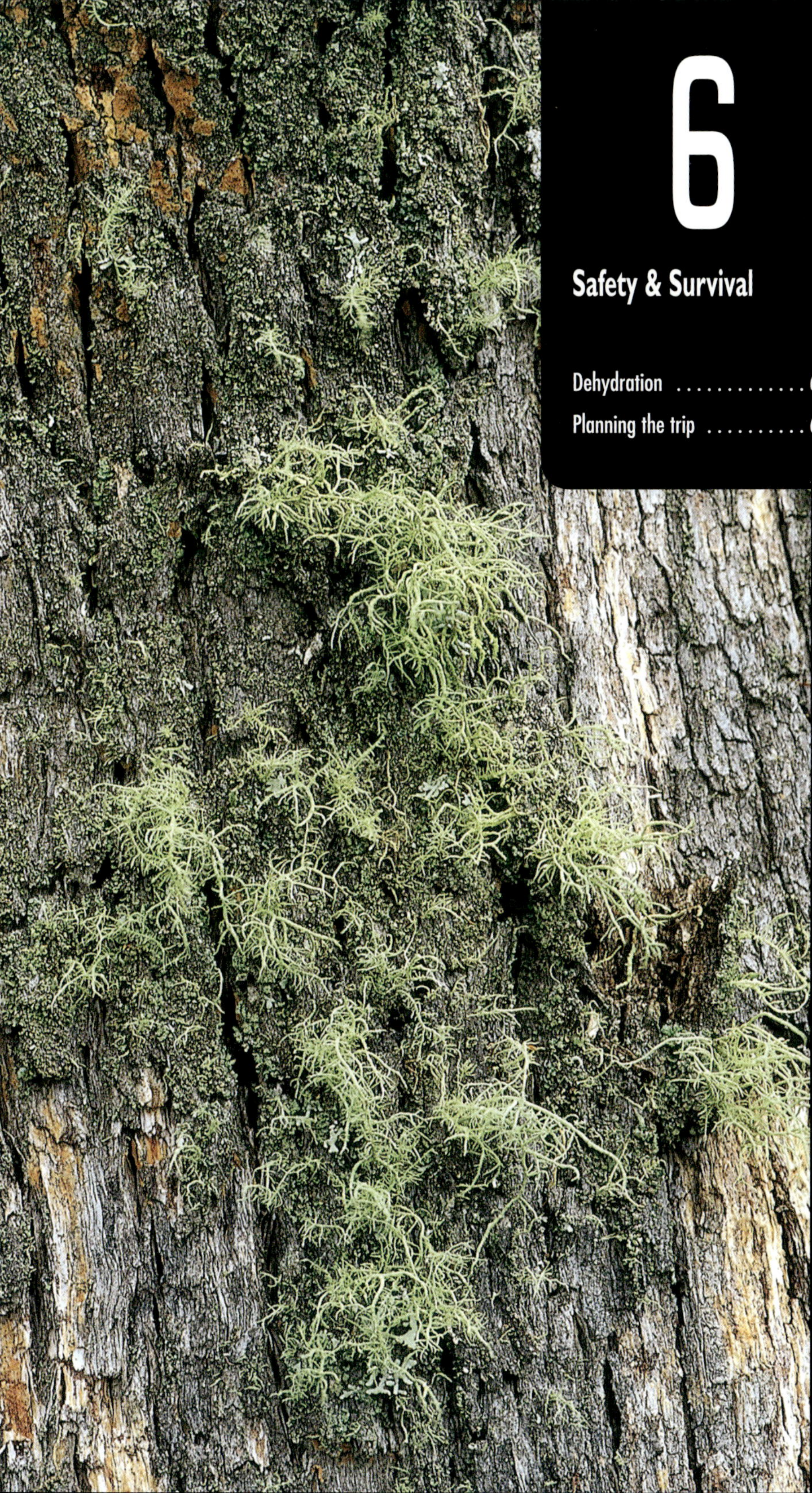

A human being has several basic needs—warmth, shelter, food, fluids, and contact with other human beings. This chapter discusses some of these needs in the context of remote area first aid.

An emergency situation can be managed most effectively in two phases:

1 Acute.

2 Longer-term.

The acute phase involves bringing the most severe injuries under control by the simplest possible means—for example, managing severe bleeding by asking casualty to hold the wound firmly and raise limb above level of heart. Once this phase is completed the first aider will have time to manage the situation in a calm and more thoughtful manner.

The following four-step management plan (APIE) is cyclical. Once you have carried out an evaluation, go back to the beginning, and reassess the situation.

- **Assess**—the injury, the casualty, and the entire situation; decide how to deal with it.
- **Plan**—the management, including gathering all equipment needed.
- **Implement**—carry out the management.
- **Evaluate**—has the plan achieved what you wanted it to?

Another helpful generalisation when planning the priorities of survival is the Rule of 3's which indicates the length of time a person can survive without basic needs:

RULE OF 3's			
3 minutes without oxygen	30 hours without shelter	3 days without water	30 days without food

Dehydration

People generally need more water in a survival situation than in any other situation. Whether in the desert, sea or even snow, the body requires more water when outdoors. Dehydration is one of the most prevalent conditions in a survival situation, and must be avoided. Feeling thirsty is in fact a late sign of needing to drink more!

Dehydration is a consequence of losing more fluid than is being taken into the body. Due to this disruption of fluid balance urine collects in the bladder more slowly and, because the urine contains less water, has a higher concentration of waste products, giving it a darker yellow colour than usual. This is a warning sign that the body is becoming dehydrated, with a reduction in blood volume causing the blood to become concentrated. Another sign of dehydration is that the cells of the body, which are normally plump and round, begin to sag. When skin is pinched, it takes several seconds to resume its normal position.

To compensate for fluid loss, the person in a hot environment needs to take in more fluid than normal. Remember that by the time the casualty becomes thirsty, dehydration may be quite advanced. The average daily fluid intake for an adult in a temperate climate is about 4–6 litres per day. In a hot environment this can increase to 6–8 litres per day. The leader should not permit the group to resume activity until the casualty reports that the urine is clear or a pale straw colour.

The theory of 'rationing your sweat, not your water' is important. This means drinking to maintain the lowest level of dehydration possible. Water is better inside the body than inside the water bottle. To ration your sweat in hot environments, you must limit your activity during the hottest part of the day. Rest as much as possible in the most shady position available during the day. Use the cool of the morning, evening and night for activity.

It is important to remember to limit physical activity to the coolest part of the day, so as to minimise sweating. Other actions which will reduce sweating are:

- remaining fully clothed—keep clothes loose
- moving slowly
- maintaining a minimum of dehydration
- remembering APIE—plan each and every action carefully

Collecting water

Water can be obtained from many sources, though some should be avoided for fear of contamination. Information on water collection is best gained from specialist survival texts, though some suggestions are:

- condensation on grass or metal at night
- run-off from leaves
- pools in rocks or at the base of cliffs
- dew
- digging at the outside of bends in dry creeks or riverbeds
- roots, trees, vines and plants such as cactus or pigface
- solar stills
- tree-bagging—condensation forms in plastic bag placed over tree branch and foliage

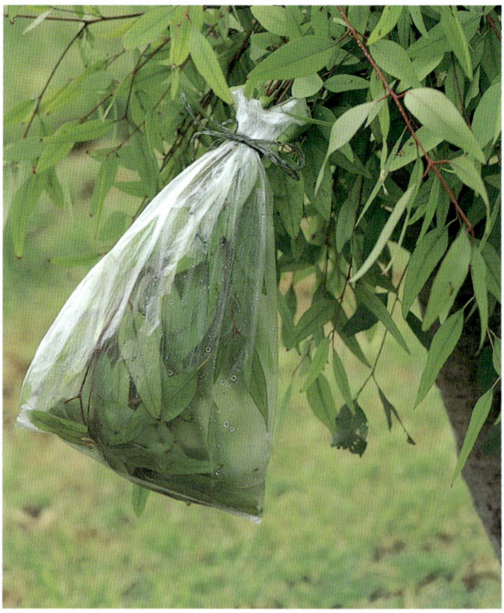

Tree-bagging

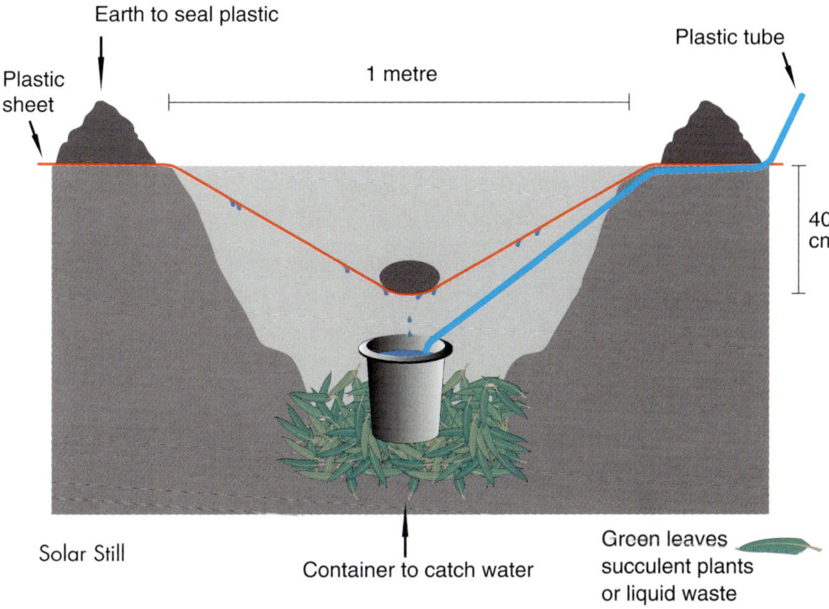

Solar Still

Do not underestimate the amount of water needed in a first aid situation. It will not only be needed for drinking and cooking, but also for hygiene, wound care and sometimes even pain relief—for example with burns.

Water should be as clear and fresh as possible for all uses; however, drinking and wound care will require the purest water you have available. Prioritising usage will require thought, care and cooperation between all party members. When planning your trip, you should consider water purification; are you going to boil, filter, or add substances to the water, such as chlorine or iodine tablets?

Planning the trip

Another important priority is that of prevention. It is always better to plan properly in order to avoid emergencies. Before heading out on a trip, always plan for the worst possible scenario and be prepared for the unforeseeable to occur. Anticipate all possible problems.

All members of the group—but particularly the leader and the first aider—should be constantly alert for the presence of danger. Use all your senses for this, including that intangible 'sixth sense'. Try to eliminate danger, not only for your group, but also for any others using the area. For example any large animal killed on the road should be moved well to the side, to prevent the next vehicle colliding with it.

All members of the group will have their own areas of responsibility, even if it is only for their own gear. It is one of the leader's responsibilities to ensure that each member takes the appropriate gear. The group should be briefed about the importance of looking out for each other, not only for emotional needs but also for the presence of danger and, for example, the signs and symptoms of hypothermia or heat exhaustion.

The leader will have many responsibilities. Some general ones are planning the trip, preparing all members (including themselves) and arranging communication—in an emergency, communication will be vital. The leader will need to be able to talk not only with the first aider and the rest of the group, but also with rescue personnel and other outside agencies. Communication skills, as well as communication devices, are important *(see ch. 5)*.

The first aider's initial responsibilities lie mainly with equipment, ensuring that all possibilities have been researched and that appropriate equipment is taken on the trip. Either the leader, the first aider or both should endeavour to gain some understanding of any potential medical problems within the group. In addition, the first aider should ensure that their first aid knowledge and practical skills are current. It may be appropriate to educate the other group members about some of the basic first aid skills which could be needed.

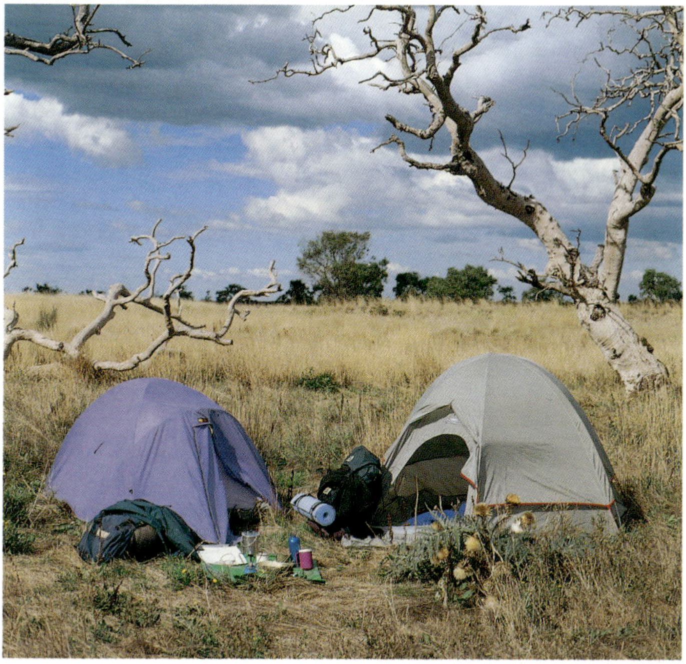

Safety and survival will depend greatly on the level of planning and preparation for the trip.

1 What equipment needs to be taken—personal and group equipment, communications, first aid items, vehicle recovery, and survival equipment?

2 Has all the appropriate equipment been gathered?

3 Is the equipment all in good order?

4 Are there several people in the group who have the knowledge and experience of how to use the equipment?

5 Is it possible—and appropriate—to improvise for any items of equipment?

It will generally not be necessary to take specialist rescue or evacuation equipment. In most parts of Australia, help will be available within a couple of days, if not a couple of hours. Rescue personnel will have the equipment and training needed to help you. Your time and resources will be best used to manage the situation where you are. Only move if you are in danger, or if you are instructed to do so—for example, moving to clearer ground so that a helicopter can more easily land. Leave evacuations and rescues to the experts.

Current communication technology may allow you to talk with the experts while in the field. Do not underestimate the value of being able to ask for advice—you may not need someone to come and get you, but it can be very reassuring to have some advice. Some of the experts you might consider contacting are:

- local hospital
- doctor—local, your own or the casualty's
- mechanic
- police
- ranger
- local residents

It may be appropriate to contact some or all of these people to advise them of your trip before leaving.

In conclusion, one of the best safety precautions to follow is to leave a trip plan with a responsible adult, along with instructions for them to follow if you do not return at the planned time. Ensure that this person will carry out your instructions.

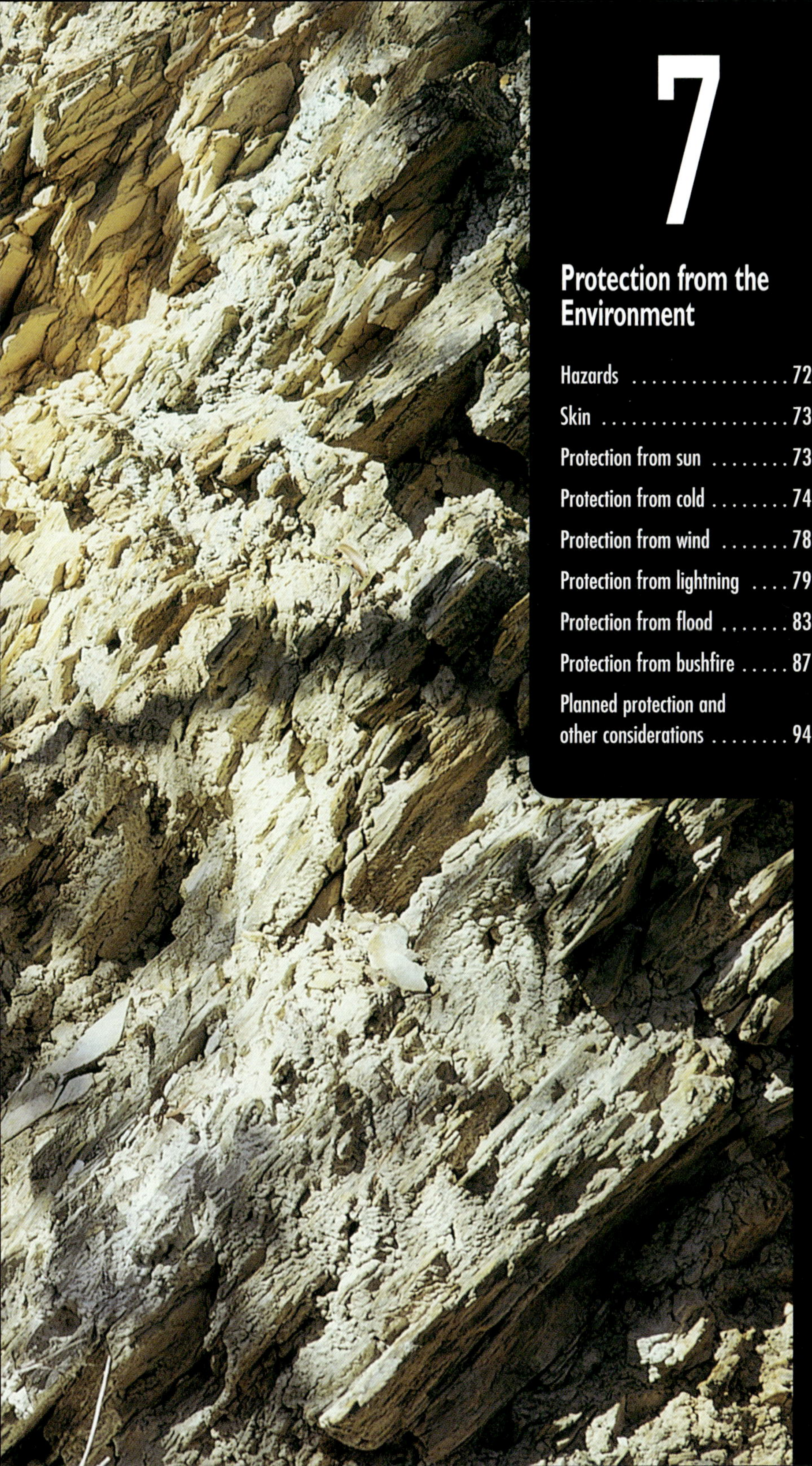

7

Protection from the Environment

Hazards

Experience has shown that most people when lost are located within 72 hours. If you become lost or stranded, location and environmental conditions can become more important than water, providing you have planned and prepared properly.

A good question to consider then is—what conditions do we need protection from?

Common hazards are overexposure to heat and cold, bites and stings, sunburn, immersion, lack of food and water, mud, dust, sand and salt. Weather conditions including sun, rain, snow, hail, lightning, wind and flood can influence the chances of survival.

Additionally, the discomfort from ailments such as a cold or the flu and problems such as a headache or an upset stomach can be as debilitating as bad sunburn and insect bites. Some of these ailments may also be easily passed on to other members of the party.

On the grounds that 'prevention is better than cure' try to avoid exposure by planning well in advance for trips during times of weather extremes. Try to find out as much as possible about the area where the trip is taking place.

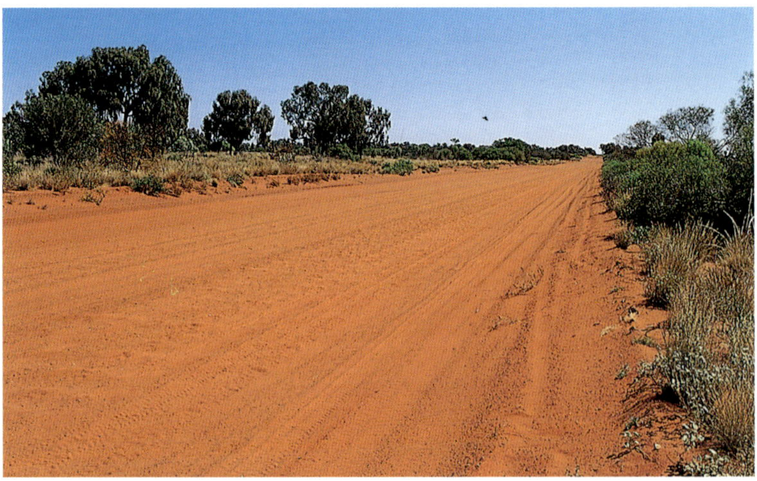

Skin

Our skin acts as a barrier between ourselves and the external world. It provides efficient and effective heating, cooling, insulation, waterproofing and sensation and can adapt to a changing environment. Being almost waterproof, it prevents rapid absorption and evaporation and thereby helps keep the amount of water in our body constant. It assists in shielding against injury and usually heals quickly. Probably the most complex of its functions is to help maintain a constant internal body temperature.

Protection from sun

One of the most important aspects of travel almost anywhere in Australia at any time of the year is the need for shelter. In hot desert climates an active person needs to replace up to 6 to 8 litres of water daily. In an emergency it is usually much more productive to take measures to reduce body fluid loss rather than try to find or produce drinkable water. This basically means trying to conserve sweat, particularly in the hot parts of the day, by minimising activity and staying in the shade as much as possible. Temporary shelters for this purpose might include:

- space blanket from the first aid kit—placed over, underneath or behind the person
- umbrella
- natural shelter such as cliffs, large rocks or vegetation
- shade from vehicle—either beside or underneath, or from open car boot or bonnet
- aircraft wing
- makeshift 'lean-to' or 'A-frame' shelter—but be aware that these take longer to build than might be expected
- bed that sits 30 cm above the ground can reduce the temperature by up to 10°C

The most important shelter, however, will be provided by clothing. Serious consideration should be given to wearing shirts which cover the back of the neck, long pants, hat, sunglasses and footwear. Clothing will also provide significant protection against bites from insects and snakes. Sunscreen is important to prevent sunburn.

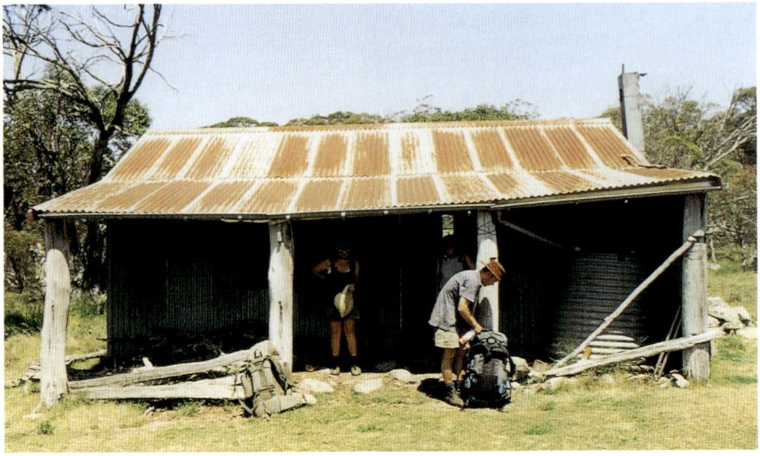

Protection from cold

Outback travellers should be aware that a hot day may well be followed by a cold night, with temperatures dropping near to or below freezing. South-east Australia has large areas where prolonged periods of cold weather are normal every autumn, winter and spring.

Australian Bureau of Meteorology figures show average July minimum temperatures of 3°C or lower over a vast area, from Toowoomba in southern Queensland, south and then west to Ballarat in Victoria. Virtually all of Tasmania is also in this category. About one third of this area experiences winter snowfall and most areas above 1300–1400 m elevation are snow-covered for extended periods.

Much of the terrain in these areas is remarkably rugged, even though in international terms, the hills and mountains are not high. Visibility from ground level may be obscured and orientation difficult even in good weather. Small towns are widely scattered throughout the region.

In addition to low temperatures, windchill is an important factor. Wind velocity is consistently higher at higher altitudes. These conditions increase in winter months. Snow also increases in these months, although it may fall at any time of year, causing loss of visibility and other problems. Loss of body heat caused by these conditions may cause health problems.

How the body loses heat

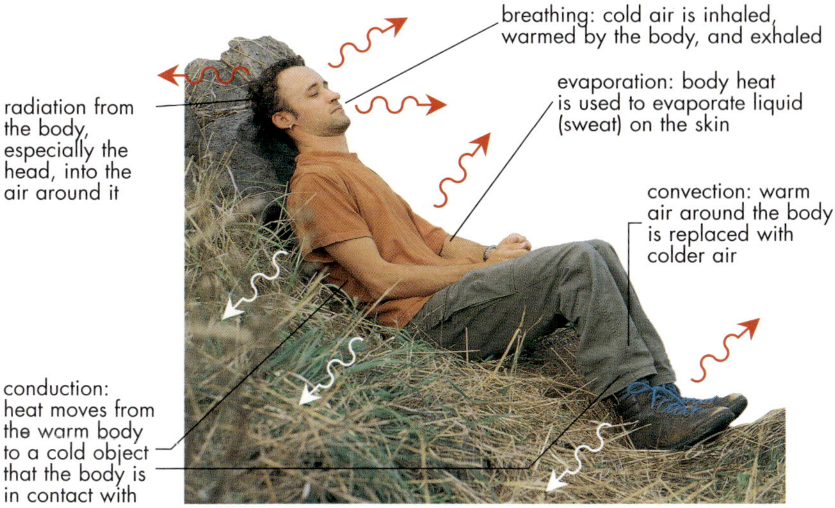

Climatic conditions may vary greatly. Temperatures in the mountains can fall below 0°C in any month of the year. This is not necessarily associated with precipitation. Apart from monthly variability, there can be very rapid change in daily patterns. Experienced locals can often predict such changes, but there is no guarantee of safety. A minor injury combined with sudden foul weather could prove fatal. In less than an hour conditions may change from clear to a severe blizzard. Being prepared is vital. Always remember:

1 You will not be found easily in a blizzard.

2 You put other people at risk if you become lost.

3 You may become lost when only hundreds of metres from civilisation.

Note: Always inform someone of your intended destination, route and time of return.

Ultraviolet light exposure is increased at altitude especially when mountain skies are smog free. Light intensity is magnified by reflection off snow and water by up to 90%. Sunburn and eye burns are hazards of clear, bright mountain weather.

In cold climates it is important to shelter from wind and rain to reduce or eliminate the windchill factor. Sheltering inside a vehicle will be more effective in the cold.

Clothing

Correct clothing, including adequate footwear, becomes potentially a life saving measure in cold climates. It is generally sound advice to wear three distinct layers consisting of undergarments, a foundation layer and the outer or protective layer. Retention of temperature and removal of moisture should be considered when selecting underwear. Be aware that cotton can lose up to 90% of its insulating capacity when wet whereas wool loses only 50%. Protection of head, neck and hands is essential. Use a beanie, scarf and gloves or mittens, with good sunglasses or goggles being important additions in snow. The outer or protective layer should be windproof yet able to 'breathe'.

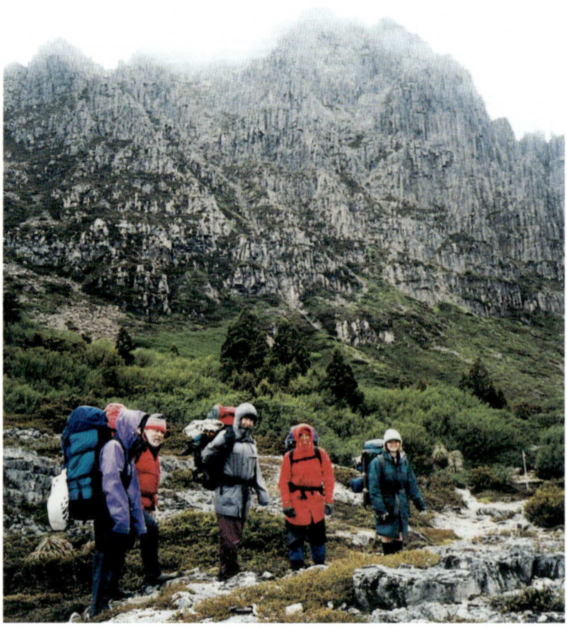

Fire

Fire is an important resource when caught out in the cold as it cooks, sterilises, warms and acts as a signal when necessary. It is wise to always carry some form of fire starter on trips—such as waterproof matches or a lighter. Ensure that the fire is started away from the party or vehicle and move closer to it when safe to do so. If no matches or lighter are available, then, on a vehicle trip, the cigarette lighter can be used to ignite a petrol-soaked rag. Other methods, such as using the spark from a car battery or even a torch battery, are potentially dangerous and less controllable. Advice should be sought as part of trip preparation.

Hail

Shelter from the more violent elements such as hail should generally be an emergency, short-term measure and to a large extent it is 'everyone for themselves'. Any obvious natural shelter should be utilised and it may be appropriate to crouch down with a pack over your head. In any party trapped in the open, adults may be able to use their own bodies to provide temporary protection for children. The first aider should check the party for any injuries before proceeding—at least ice for soft tissue injuries should not be a problem.

Snow

Any trip into the snow should be prepared for properly. Snow can occur at any time of the year in south-east Australia. If caught out, immediate action is required to take shelter from the wind and snow, ensuring appropriate cover underneath as well as above each person. This should be quickly followed by an assessment of the nourishment needs and capabilities of the group.

In most instances building a temporary shelter such as an igloo will consume too much time, and walking groups or similar parties in particular may not be equipped for such activities. On the other hand it may well be possible to dig out a simple wall in the snow to shelter from the wind in an exposed area. Otherwise, normal and sensible precautions to reduce the possibility of hypothermia should be taken. It is extremely important that not only the first aider, but the whole party, is sufficiently well-educated in recognising the initial onset of problems relating to the cold.

A blizzard combining snow and wind can pose significant problems and risks, and immediate shelter, keeping the whole party together, is essential.

Protection from wind

Probably one of the most important elements from which to shelter is the wind. It introduces a new array of potential problems including sand, dust, salt, dehydration, burning, windchill and flying debris. In an emergency, shelter becomes the single most important consideration of all because strong winds can blow for days.

Many makeshift shelters including some tents will not be adequate. A more permanent shelter will be necessary. In the short term, using a coat or space blanket and crouching down will provide immediate relief while the party gathers its wits, assesses the situation and plans what action to take.

Natural shelters such as cliffs and large rocks or boulders will also help, as long as there is safe access to and exit from the leeward side. Vehicles and buildings can also provide adequate shelter in most instances. If not, hopefully the party will be able to contact the local emergency services to seek advice and assistance. This aspect also highlights the necessity of maintaining contact throughout the trip with someone who can provide weather updates and to whom your situation can be reported. Vehicles and boats should be parked facing into the wind—if visibility is poor and safety is a concern then the lights should be left on during this time (be careful not to flatten battery).

Prolonged exposure to high winds in an emergency can often mean there will be difficulties in constructing a more permanent shelter for eating and sleeping. A combination of teamwork, APIE (assess, plan, implement, evaluate)—when the group will be familiar with their own equipment as well as the current situation—and 'brainstorming' (assessment and planning) will resolve most problems. For example, while camping, a series of tent flies can often be made more secure than a tent at the expense of absolute wind-, water-, and dust-proofing.

A combination of wind and a cold environment brings additional hazards because more long-term shelter and active warming both need to be considered as high priorities.

Protection from lightning

Lightning is the electrical discharge produced when differences in ground and atmospheric electrical charge are large enough to overcome the insulating effect of air. Lightning strikes may occur within clouds, between clouds, or between clouds and the ground. Thunder is the sound produced by the explosive expansion of air heated by the lightning strike.

Lightning is usually associated with heavy rain. However, in northern Australia, 'dry' thunderstorms are quite common.

We see lightning at the instant it occurs, but thunder travels much more slowly as the speed of sound is much slower than the speed of light. This enables us to determine how far away the thunderstorm is. Sound takes about 3 seconds to travel a kilometre. Therefore to estimate the distance in kilometres, count the seconds between a lightning flash and the thunder, and divide by three.

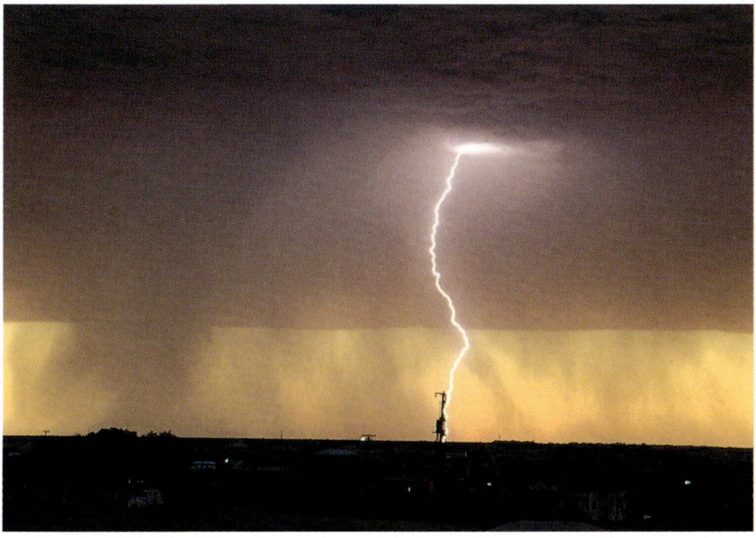

People may be burnt and electrocuted, either by being hit directly by lightning, or more commonly by electrical currents in the ground or other objects resulting from a lightning strike.

After lightning strikes, electrical currents travel through the earth following the path of least electrical resistance. Least resistance may be offered by wire fences and railway tracks, and by moist conditions.

The aim is to avoid being caught in the least safe locations—remember that nowhere is really safe. The safest locations are inside houses, large buildings and all metal vehicles including caravans. Fabric tents offer no protection and small sheds offer uncertain protection.

If outside, avoid presenting a target to the lightning by ensuring your body does not project above the surrounding landscape. Avoid the tops of hills and ridges, flat open country, beaches and water. Also avoid items that present targets to lightning such as isolated trees.

Whether inside or in the open, avoid items that might conduct lightning currents to you from a distance, e.g. metal and electrical equipment.

In the open, a small boat, fabric tent or small shed

1 Crouch down with your feet together and hands around your knees.

2 Insulate yourself from the ground if possible by crouching on some insulating material such as a foam pad, coiled rope, rucksack (no steel frame), folded dry clothes, or a small loose rock. If wearing footwear with metal reinforcing, remove.

3 **DO NOT** lie down as this greatly increases the chances that a ground current will pass through your body.

4 Remove metal objects from hair and head covering.

5 If in a group in the open, keep at least 10 metres apart so that if a person is injured, others can render first aid.

Inside buildings

1 Close all doors and windows and stay away from windows.

2 Avoid fireplaces, plumbing and steel beams as these may conduct lightning.

3 Avoid using telephones, two-way radios and other electrical appliances as these may conduct lightning.

In a vehicle

All metal vehicles are safe as they act as a 'Faraday cage or shield'—the area within the vehicle is shielded from outside electricity.

1 **DO NOT** touch the sides, roof, floor or bare metal parts of the vehicle as these may carry lightning current.

2 Close windows and doors.

Vehicles with fabric, fibreglass or other non-metal roofs or sides are not safe. In particular, get away from vehicles without metal cabs, such as tractors, bulldozers, beach buggies, golf carts, motorcycles and bicycles.

On water

1 If swimming or boating, get out of and away from open water.

2 If caught in a small boat, go below deck if possible. Otherwise crouch as described above.

3 In a small boat seek shelter near a tall object such as a jetty or a bridge.

Note: Boats with steel hulls and superstructure will protect you in the same way as a car, provided you are below deck.

In the bush or a forest

1 Avoid tall trees.

2 Seek shelter in low areas under a thick growth of small trees or scrub.

Note: If tall trees cannot be avoided, seek shelter just beyond the spread of the foliage.

In hilly or mountainous country

A convex slope is more prone to direct lightning strike than a level or concave slope, but ground currents pose serious dangers even in apparently safe places. This is especially so in rocky areas because the lightning currents are more likely to travel along the surface of the rock as it offers less electrical resistance. The risk is increased if the area is wet or the rock mineralised.

1 Crouch down on a level or concave area of an open slope, at least 2 metres from any cliff or large rock.

   Note: The zone of protection from direct lightning strikes at the base of a rock wall 20 m high is between 2–20 m from the cliff.

2 Ensure your body does not project above the landscape—move off ridges, hilltops.

3 Avoid sheltering in narrow vertical gullies, small holes or caves or overhanging rock.

   Note: In such locations, the body may act as a bridge for the current path. Deep dry caves are safer, but insulate yourself from the rock.

In open country

1 Crouch down and seek shelter in dry ravines, valleys or low spots where the ground is concave.

2 Be aware of the flash flood potential.

3 Avoid presenting a target to the lightning by ensuring your body does not project from the surrounding landscape.

4 Avoid objects which might act as lightning targets such as tall isolated trees, power poles, overhead wires, wire fences, metal pipes, railway tracks, and other metallic paths which could carry lightning to you from a distance.

5 **DO NOT** ride horses, and stay away from tractors and other farm and sporting equipment which may attract lightning.

After the storm

Those injured by lightning will not carry electrical charge and will be quite safe to touch.

1 Follow DRABC—perform CPR if necessary.

2 Manage burns *(see p. 162)*.

3 Arrange medical attention for those who appear temporarily stunned but otherwise unhurt, as they may have internal injuries.

4 Remain alert for flash floods and other hazards associated with severe weather.

Protection from flood

Flooding, severe storm and lightning may be experienced anywhere and at any time in Australia.

Important factors in flood safety and damage include:

- flood water depth
- water current
- amount of mud and other material carried by the water
- safe wading depth, which decreases rapidly as current increases
- objects such as broken glass and splintered wood in the water
- how much warning time you have to prepare for the flood and/or to be safely evacuated

Causes of injury

Most of the deaths from flooding in Australia result from people driving or walking through floodwaters. Floodwater depth and current are easily misjudged. In small streams, the water level may change suddenly. Some deaths have resulted from people camping in dry riverbeds.

It is likely that many of those thought to have drowned in floods, especially 'flash floods', may actually have been killed by the violence of the water, or as a result of striking objects in the water or the riverbed. Being a good swimmer in this case may not help.

Note: DO NOT enter floodwaters, especially where an obvious current exists.

Other injuries from floodwaters include:

- risk of becoming ill after drinking water polluted by sewage—water in urban areas and many recreation areas and national parks can become polluted with human waste during flooding
- being injured by objects in the floodwater—broken glass, torn metal, splintered timber and electrical wires
- injuries from vehicle accidents caused by road washouts
- electrocution by overhead powerlines—in boats on floodwater, be aware of powerlines, as they may be dangerously close to aerials or masts

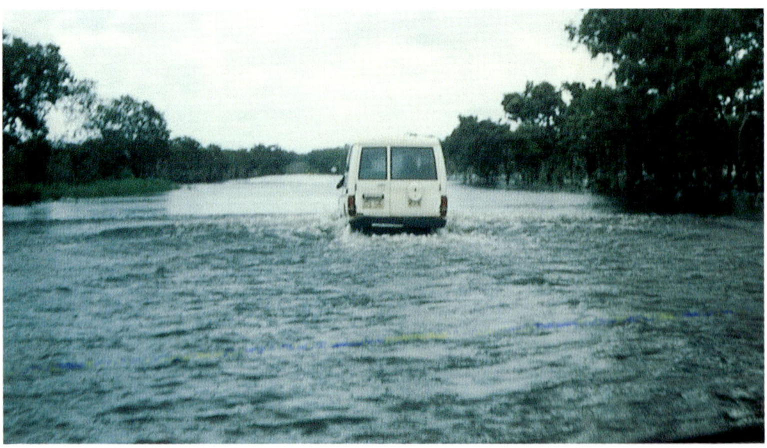

Warnings

News warnings are provided for flooding in remote areas, rivers and streams. Weather forecasts will indicate the likelihood of flooding by forecasting heavy rain or thunderstorms. In the outback, floodwaters may take several weeks or even months to travel from the area of rain.

People need to be aware of the environmental indicators of flooding, which include:

- continuous heavy rain
- thunderstorm activity in the area
- the roaring sound of an approaching flash flood
- cyclones

If living or staying in an area for an extended period, find out about the local flood history and the safe (high ground) areas.

Types of flooding

- sea—strong wind and waves can raise the sea above its normal level, by as much as several metres; especially dangerous if this occurs at high tide; tropical and subtropical Australia are most at risk; if abnormal or dangerously high tides are forecast, leave the area and head inland to high ground—seek shelter from accompanying high winds
- major inland rivers—Warrego, Paroo and Murray–Darling system; warnings are usually given days or even months in advance
- normally dry rivers and creeks in arid and semi-arid Australia—often flash flooding with strong currents and virtually no warning; this is particularly dangerous as flooding may occur very rapidly in areas that are deceptively dry, well-vegetated and do not look like riverbeds—never camp in dry riverbeds (check with locals)
- urban runoff after storms—urban drainage channels and streams are very dangerous as water levels rise and fall rapidly
- dam bursts—farm and mining dams pose the greatest risk of bursting; generally there are no warnings; however, in most cases, sustained heavy rain would precede failure—avoid camping below farm and mining dams, or near streams below these dams

Actions to take before flooding

Taking the actions outlined below will help minimise the risks of, and damage caused by, flooding.

1 Avoid camping at the bottom of gullies and in dry riverbeds, especially during the wet season in northern Australia (November to April).

2 Listen to weather forecasts—have a battery-powered radio with spare batteries; if this fails, use the car radio.

3 Be aware of the environmental indicators of flooding.

4 Know the relationship between flood heights and the height of your location, so that you can interpret warnings.

5 Move belongings and animals above the estimated flood height.

6 Remove or protect machinery by sealing vulnerable sections with sandbags.

7 Ensure chemicals and fuel supplies are stored securely above flood height.

8 Evacuate early if you plan to leave—it is dangerous to evacuate late.

9 **DO NOT** attempt to cross rivers or streams just before flooding as the water may rise suddenly.

Note: Evacuating from stable buildings and other relatively safe places at the last moment is dangerous, because transport routes are usually flooded first.

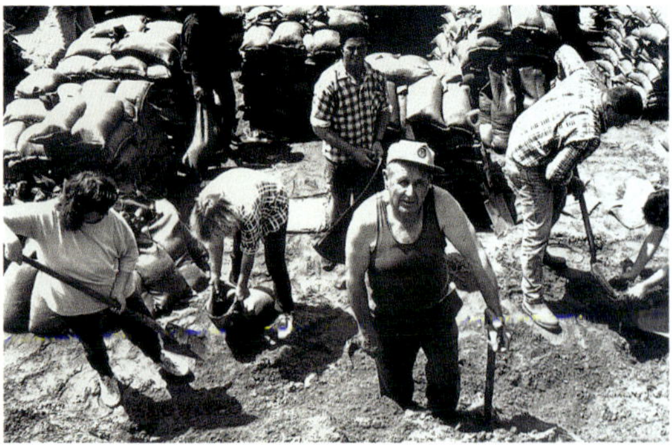

During and after the flood

1 If caught in a narrow valley by a flash flood—climb up the valley sides.

2 If driving along the bottom of the valley—abandon your vehicle and climb on foot.

3 Monitor weather forecasts.

4 Sterilise the water either chemically or by boiling before drinking as it may be polluted.

5 Watch out for other refugees from the flood such as snakes.

6 Avoid entering any floodwater either by foot or in a vehicle.

7 **DO NOT** attempt to cross fast-moving flooded streams by boat, foot or vehicle.

Note: Do not enter water if it is swirling, flowing fast, contains floating logs, or if you can hear stones rolling along the riverbed. Water is usually most dangerous at river bends and the current may be too fast to cross safely in the straight, shallow sections.

8 Be aware of overhead powerlines—the depth of floodwater may make them much closer than normal.

9 If in a car—once a safe crossing spot is found, remove the fan belt and cover the distributor—proceed slowly and steadily.

Note: Dry out brakes by applying light pressure on the brake pedal as you drive, until grip returns.

Protection from bushfire

Each year in Australia bushfires, which have the ability to travel swiftly over hundreds of kilometres of bushland, cause severe loss of property. Occasionally lives are also lost. Fear of fire is one of humanity's greatest fears. Unreasoned panic has often led to death when comparative safety has been nearby. Knowledge of some simple but effective rules can help you stay alive in a bushfire or grassfire.

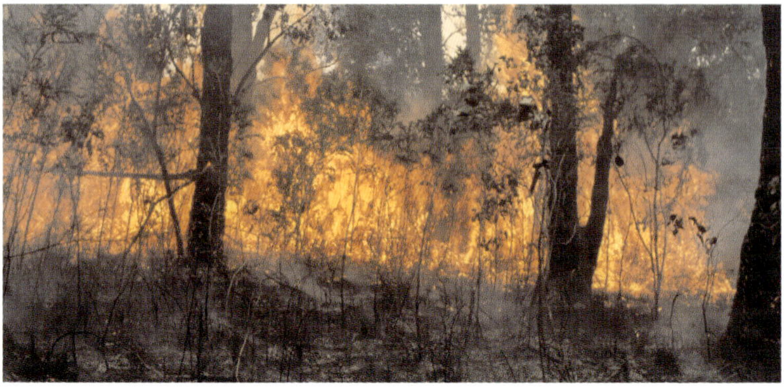

The fire triangle

Three elements—fuel, air and heat—are necessary to have fire. Remove any of these and the fire will go out.

1 If clothing is alight, remove air by covering the person in a wool blanket and rolling them on ground.

2 Apply water to fire to reduce heat and displace air with steam.

3 Clear an area around a campfire to deprive fire of fuel.

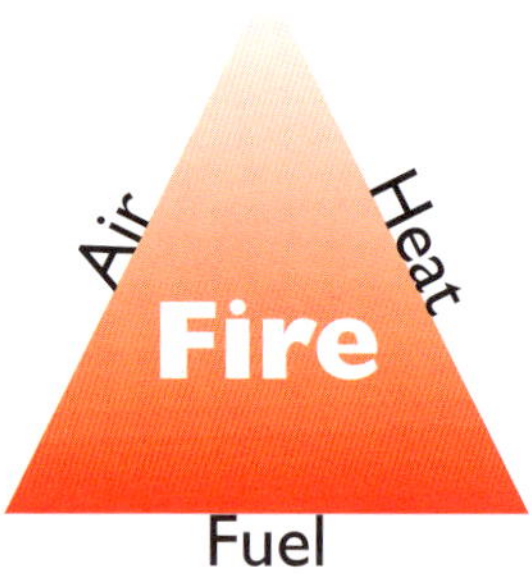

Wind-borne heat

Air is heated as the wind blows a fire forward. Hot air tends to heat objects in advance of the fire. Heat felt in the air is an immediate indication that a fire is very close. Take safety precautions before the arrival of the fire.

Radiated heat

Radiated heat is one source of danger in a bushfire. Few people are actually burnt to death in bushfires. The majority die from radiated heat before the flames reach them. The temperature of a low intensity fire will be about 1000°C, and the heat level rises sharply as fire intensity increases.

Protection from radiated heat is a major factor in bushfire survival. Any measure of protection—e.g. rolling in mud—is preferable to serious burn or radiation injury or death.

Note: Radiation travels in straight lines—it does not travel around corners. Radiation will not pass through solid barriers such as house walls or earth banks, but it can pass through glass.

Trapped by bushfire

You may become trapped by bushfire when you are:

- on foot
- in a vehicle
- in a building with little or no cleared area of protection facing the fire

DO NOT panic—you must remain calm and assess your position logically.

The actions listed below will minimise danger.

1 If possible go to an area that is already burnt or free of fuel.

2 **DO NOT** attempt to run through a fire front, or climb into water tanks as this water heats rapidly.

3 Seek shelter—in a creek, dam or waterhole at the side furthest from the fire.

4 If no water is available, hide behind a raised object—a log, rock or tree stump—in a fuel-free clearing.

5 Seek shelter away from any potential fuel and cover any exposed skin with dirt or clothing.

6 In bare areas, hollows in the ground—e.g. wheel ruts—provide some protection.

7 If a harnessed animal is involved, remove the harness and let the animal run free.

8 If possible, lie face down with feet towards the oncoming fire.

In a vehicle

If caught in a fire while in a vehicle follow the steps below.

1 Stay in the car and do not try to run—the main intensity of the fire will pass quickly.

2 **DO NOT** attempt to drive through thick smoke.

3 Stop the vehicle on bare ground—e.g. on a road.

4 Turn off the ignition and switch on headlights and hazard lights.

5 Wind up all windows and close all vents.

6 Stay below the level of windows.

7 Shelter from radiant heat by lying on the floor and covering yourself with woollen blankets, floor mats or clothing.

8 Remain in the car until the fire front has passed—even if the tyres are burning. The petrol tank is unlikely to explode.

9 If you have to get out of the car at any time, remember to cover all exposed skin areas and move to burnt ground.

10 Toxic gases from upholstery may make it necessary for you to leave your vehicle despite the danger.

Note: If it becomes too hot to remain in the car, it will be even hotter outside and therefore extremely dangerous. Use all resources available—e.g. water, extra clothing, woollen blankets—to enable you to stay in the car.

In a building

The actions listed below will reduce danger inside a building.

1 Dress in protective clothing made of natural materials such as wool or cotton—avoid synthetics.

2 Be aware that spot fires may start on the roof or other parts of the building—someone should be outside for as long as possible to watch for spot fires.

3 If time permits, block the roof downpipes and fill the gutters with water.

4 Remove flammable items from against house—e.g. doormats, blinds, outdoor furniture.

5 Move inside the building— close all doors and windows, and block all gaps beneath doors with wet towels or blankets.

6 Remove curtains (unless they are woollen) and move all furniture away from windows.

7 Fill all utensils, baths and sinks with water. Soak blankets, towels and bags for use as fire beaters or protective covering.

8 Watch for embers and be ready to douse spot fires inside.

9 If absolutely necessary shelter in the part of the building furthest from the fire.

10 Remember that the coolest and cleanest air is near the floor.

11 The main fire will pass in about 5 minutes—during the next 30 minutes, the building will be at greatest risk so monitor closely.

12 Search for fires with care—inspect the roof and other areas where debris is smouldering.

13 If the building is alight and you are unable to extinguish the blaze—cover all exposed skin and move to a burnt out area.

14 Stay in the vicinity of the building—firefighters need to know where you are.

Remember:

- main danger is radiant heat from bushfires
- if fighting fire or trapped by fire—wear full-length garments, preferably made from wool or cotton (not synthetics)
- remain calm—do not panic
- never try to run through a fire front
- air temperature near the ground is relatively cool and there is likely to be sufficient oxygen to breathe and survive
- use a wet handkerchief over the mouth and nose to prevent smoke inhalation
- over 90% of bushfires occur because people light them—take care with campfires and don't throw lighted cigarettes out of car windows while travelling
- avoid bushfires unless you are personally involved—your curiosity could cost your life and the lives of others
- obey all directions given to you by the emergency services—e.g. fire and police officers

Preventing bushfires

People living in areas prone to bushfires need to take the precautions listed below before the bushfire season begins.

1 Regularly slash and mow the grass around your home to lower the fuel level.

2 Ensure that you have a reserve water supply in a nearby tank or dam, with an underground pipe to your home. This will assist firefighters in saving your home.

3 Install an outside sprinkler system, ensuring that sprays can be directed towards the roof and walls.

4 Fix window shutters.

5 Keep all flammable liquids away from the house in an enclosed shed.

6 Remove potential fuel from around house; consider low fire risk planting.

7 Make sure your roof is well-sealed to avoid spark entry.

8 Keep guttering clear of leaves and other build-up of flammable material.

Note: Fire services have more information on bushfire precautions and procedures. If you live in an area prone to bushfires, seek information from these authorities.

Camping

Select a campsite near a creek or waterfall. However, never camp in dry creekbeds as these can flash flood. A good water supply can be useful in fighting a bushfire and can also be used as a safe refuge. If water is not available, then select a site with good access and escape routes. Make sure you know exactly where clearings, creeks and roads are in the vicinity of your camp.

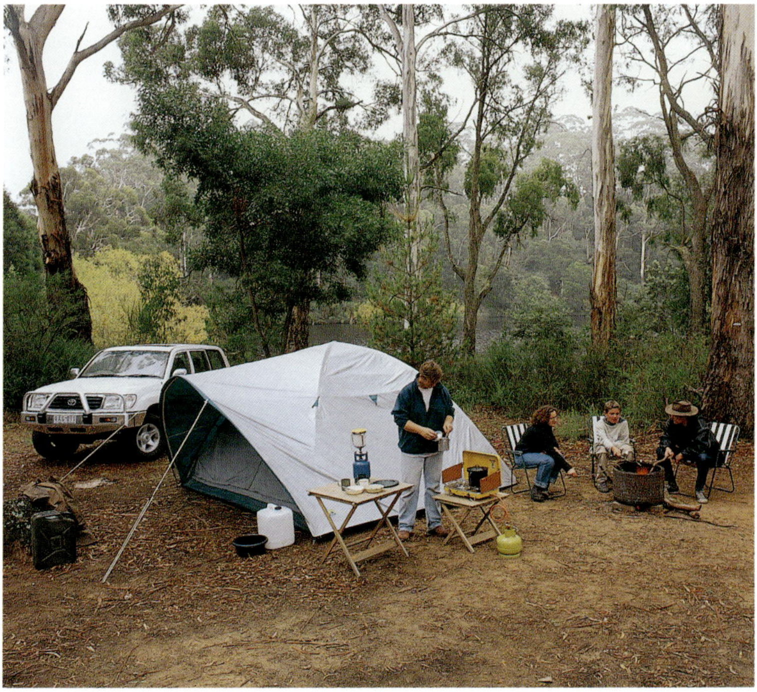

Clear an area around your campsite of all flammable material, such as leaves, wood and bark. This can act as a firebreak and increases fire safety. Remember that a tidy camp is a safer camp. Do not leave papers, cartons and other rubbish lying around—use a rubbish container.

When making a cooking fire, use a pit. Never leave the fire unattended. In some states, it is an offence to leave an open fire unattended. Before leaving the camp, ensure that the fire is completely extinguished.

Never use candles or other open flames inside a tent. If the tent should catch fire, evacuate it immediately and then collapse it—adjoining tents should also be evacuated and collapsed.

When travelling in remote areas, it is wise to check with local authorities on camping requirements. Do not be the one to start a bushfire—learn bushfire sense and live.

Planned protection and other considerations

By working our way through all of the problems that might occur in an emergency, we will be able to plan to prevent them happening in the first place.

The qualities of an ideal campsite might include the following:

- good access and escape routes
- good toilet facilities—sanitary considerations
- near a creek or waterfall—not in a dry creekbed
- natural shelter such as a cliff or high bank
- on higher ground than the surroundings, but not the highest point
- shaded, but be aware of risk of falling limbs or trees

Listed below are some additional aspects of protection in remote areas of Australia.

1 The 'Rule of Threes' suggests that for any trip there should always be enough water for everyone for at least three days under adverse conditions *(see p. 65)*—possibly up to 8 litres per person per day. This is particularly important towards the end of the trip when food and water stocks are getting low.

2 It is important to maintain contact with the adult responsible for putting into action agreed emergency procedures, especially as the trip draws to an end.

3 The importance of adequate clothing for protection from the weather or from insects and snakes cannot be over-emphasised.

4 All assessment and planning have to be put into proper perspective for the trip concerned. Any and all of the considerations noted in this chapter will vary in priority depending on such things as the terrain to be covered—bushy, open, hilly, flat—and planned duration and type of trip—day at the beach, multi-day walk or vehicle-based. Even so, it is common for leaders of one day walking trips to carry a pack containing sufficient supplies for several days. This is considered a good way of anticipating and coping with any emergencies.

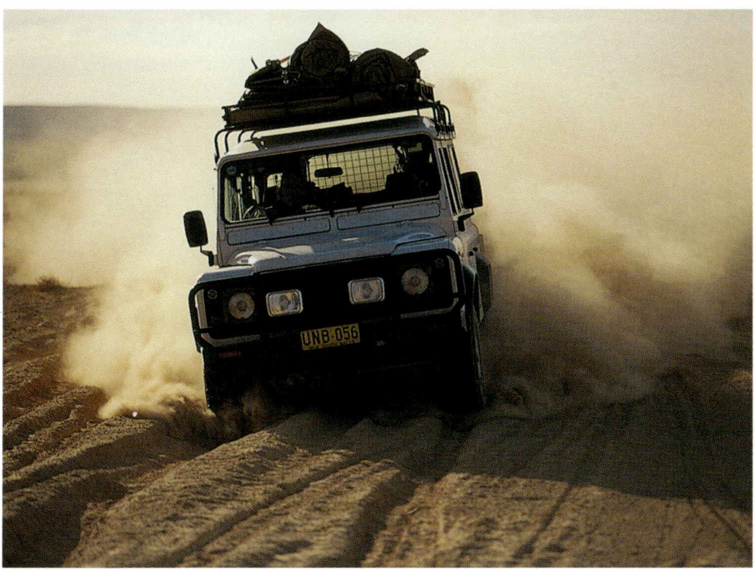

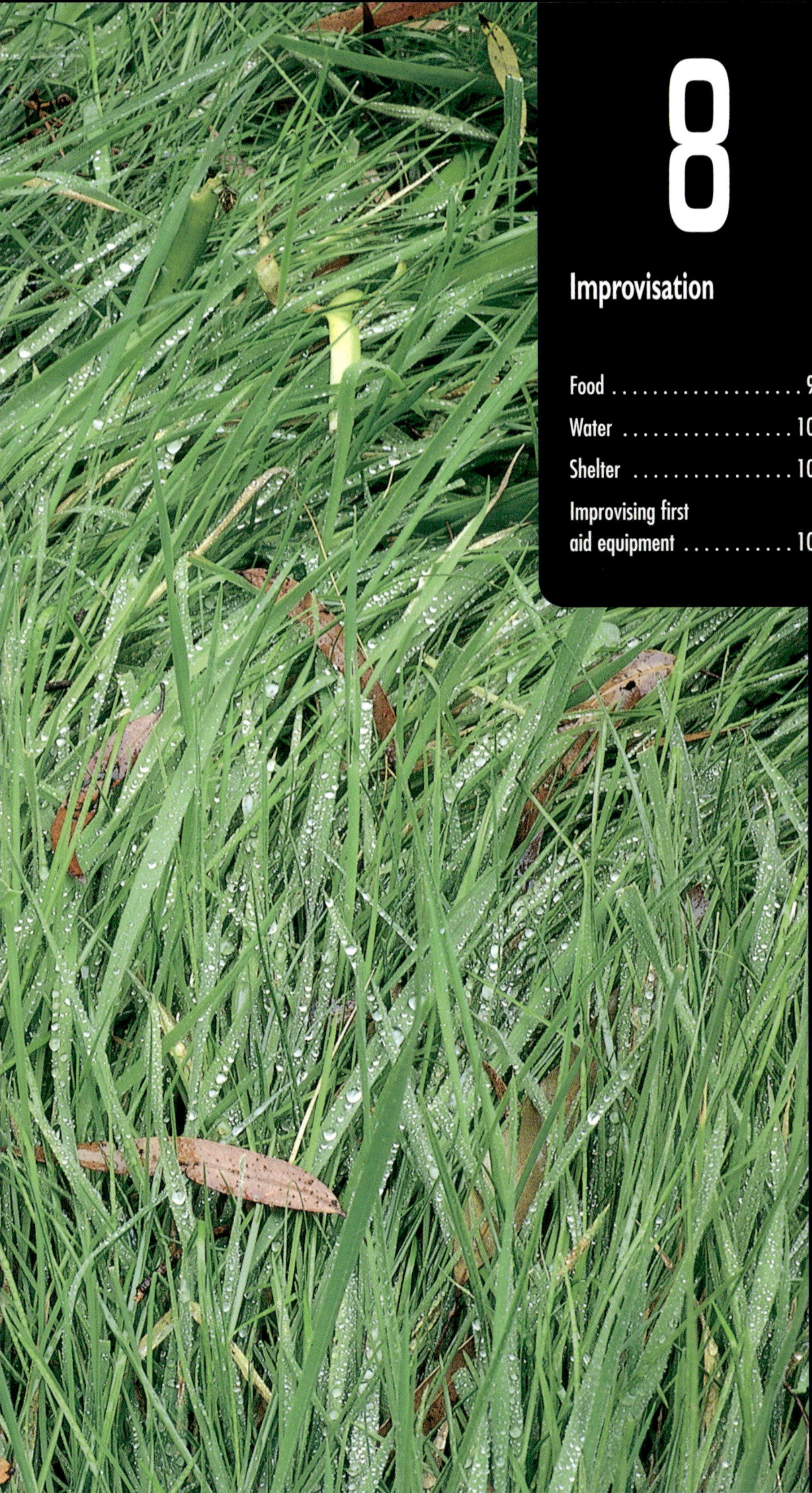

8

Improvisation

Any attempt to use improvised materials in a remote area for any purpose requires careful consideration. Use of the memory aid APIE (assess, plan, implement, evaluate) is again appropriate for first aid as well as most other activities.

As an example let us apply APIE to the construction of an improvised stretcher.

1 Assess need to move casualty.

2 If a decision is made to move casualty, plan when and where this will take place.

3 A second group should collect suitable materials to construct the stretcher.

4 Ensure these materials will not be required for other purposes.

5 Plan how the stretcher will be made, and construct it.

6 Test the stretcher for suitability prior to loading casualty.

A decision to transport a casualty on a stretcher needs a great deal of consideration. It is really only practical to carry an adult for a short distance unless via vehicle or with at least two teams of six carriers—and even then for only a few hundred metres.

Food

The easiest way to avoid a food shortage is to plan food needs carefully. At a personal level this means that for vehicle-based desert trips in outback Australia, sufficient food should be taken for at least three days in excess the planned journey. This excess can be recycled for the next trip. In addition to this, take an 'emergency only' food supply, sufficient for at least one week. This emergency supply should consist of non-perishables such as rice, pasta, pasta sauce, self-raising flour, dried fruit and sugar, as well as a 20 litre container of water.

For trips such as walking, kayaking or canoeing, it is much more difficult to carry excess supplies, especially water, for longer journeys. In most instances the only practical solution may be to have food and water drops along the way. Even so it is usually easy for each member of the party to carry an emergency food supply sufficient for at least one day. Such items as scroggin, muesli, dried fruit and chocolate bars can provide tasty as well as nourishing food.

If you are relying on 'food off the land' to provide emergency supplies for yourself or the whole party, consider that this is not a task for the inexperienced. Therefore the following points will need to be considered.

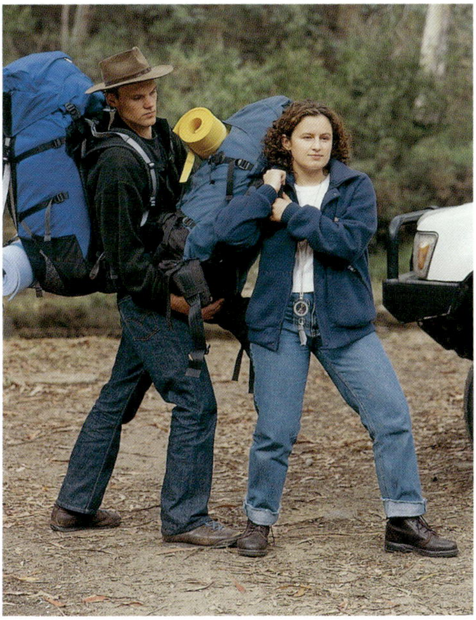

Plant food

- plant food is usually easier to get than animal food but any food requires water to aid digestion; food rationing will be a key factor in water rationing
- plant food that burns wet lips or the tongue is almost invariably poisonous to some extent
- the actual nutritional value of the plant food may be questionable
- some plants may be reasonable sources of drinkable water but it often requires considerable effort to obtain a useful quantity.

Animal food

- procuring animal food generally requires considerable skill, luck and expenditure of effort, but it has high nutritional value
- as with plant food, there is a requirement for additional water—above subsistence level—to help digestion
- while all reasonable attempts to gather food for survival will generally be acceptable, flora and fauna are protected in most parks, and firearms are prohibited

Water

Water is the primary concern for survival. Most methods for acquiring emergency water supplies in any reasonable quantity require considerable time and effort. Water obtained should be boiled for at least 10 minutes prior to consumption. With any travel into the outback or remote parts of Australia, it is advisable to thoroughly research the intended route and destination as well as the best methods of collecting water in useable amounts.

Some of the possible considerations are listed below.

Note: Always ensure that you check the quality of the water for salt and other impurities.

Creeks

- a creekbed should be easily identifiable in desert areas because of the taller vegetation following its course
- damp sand or mud may be found at the bends, either at surface level or by digging; soak a rag in the sand or mud, hand wring out the water into a container
- any exposed, live tree roots may be cut into manageable lengths and drained of their fluid early in the morning

Rocky areas

Rain usually soaks very quickly into sand or soil but can often be found up to two weeks later in depressions on rock surfaces.

Trees

The roots of several species of trees will often contain water early in the morning before the day gets too hot. Some eucalypts, wattles, boab and kurrajong trees are usually the best. The roots can be cut into lengths and the thin end placed into a container for the fluid to drain. When checking the quality, avoid any water that tastes bitter. Information about other water collection methods involving trees, such as transpiration and distillation, can be found in many good texts. The main drawback of these methods is the small return—the small quantity of water gained for significant effort required.

Other

- windmills are often built in the vicinity of underground water supplies
- if there are animal tracks nearby, you are nearly always assured of some sort of water

Purification

Sterilisation tablets work with most water sources but tend to 'taint' the resulting fluid. Substances such as iodine or chlorine tablets will also neutralise most bacteria. Using a water purifier pump is also effective.

Remember:

- it is better to try to reduce the need for water by conserving sweat and resting during the heat of the day
- conserve existing water supplies
- try to drink only in the cooler parts of the day
- ration food intake if limited water is available
- sterilise all collected water
- if feasible, even on walking trips, carry a water bottle solely for first aid purposes—minimum 500 ml but preferably 1 litre; this could also be used as an emergency supply if necessary

Shelter

It is better to prepare a shelter earlier in the day than to keep travelling until the darkness makes it difficult to move around. Guidelines on protection from the environment and making improvised and permanent shelters are detailed in chapter seven.

Improvising first aid equipment

A good guideline when reviewing and stocking a remote area first aid kit is to try, as much as possible, to carry items that can be used for more than one purpose. In this context, the following items will often be high priority and can be substituted for other purposes as listed:

- **triangular bandages**—slings, temporary bandages, constrictive bandages, constructing stretchers, securing casualty to stretcher, fracture management, padding for serious bleeding, pressure sore prevention
- **roller bandages**—sprains and strains, retaining padding, snakebite, fracture management
- **emergency accident (or 'silver foil') blanket**—hypothermia, open abdominal wounds, sucking chest wounds, windbreak (above, under or behind), signalling
- **shower cap**—retention of long hair, warming head on cold nights, hand wash basin, emergency toilet
- **sanitary napkins**—menstruation, padding larger wounds, padding splints to support fractures, pressure sore prevention
- **elastoplast dressing strip**—more versatile than adhesive strips
- **plastic bags**—washing, toilet, infectious waste, other rubbish, amputated parts, open chest and abdominal wounds, burns
- **plastic food wrap**—burns, open chest and abdominal wounds, amputations

Non first aid items

Many items carried on an expedition can also be used for improvised purposes in first aid. Always ensure before using that the items will not be required for the original or any other use, and that they are clean. Here are some items that may be able to be used for the purpose listed.

- **slings**—pantyhose, stockings, long socks, tea towels, jackets
- **roller bandages**—pantyhose, stockings, long socks, torn up T-shirt
- **emergency blanket**—tent fly, ground sheet, garbage bags
- **padding**—clothing (particularly cotton), towels, tea towels, sleeping mats (a small piece makes an excellent 'ring pad' for a blister)
- **pillows**—bulky clothing, towels
- **splints**—pack frame, ski poles, skis, newspapers, branches, maps, sleeping mats, oars

  Note: The narrower the object, the more pieces needed to make a satisfactory splint.

- **cervical collars**—newspaper, cardboard, closed cell foam (sleeping mat), hip belt from pack, towel
- **toilet**—soup tin, plastic bags, shower cap, pan, saucepan; a condom with the end cut out makes an excellent urine drain
- **stretchers**—packs, blankets, tent fly, sleeping bag, ground sheet, thermorest, skis, ski poles
- **dressing strip**—cotton clothing, electrical tape
- **washing**—shower cap, saucepan, dishes

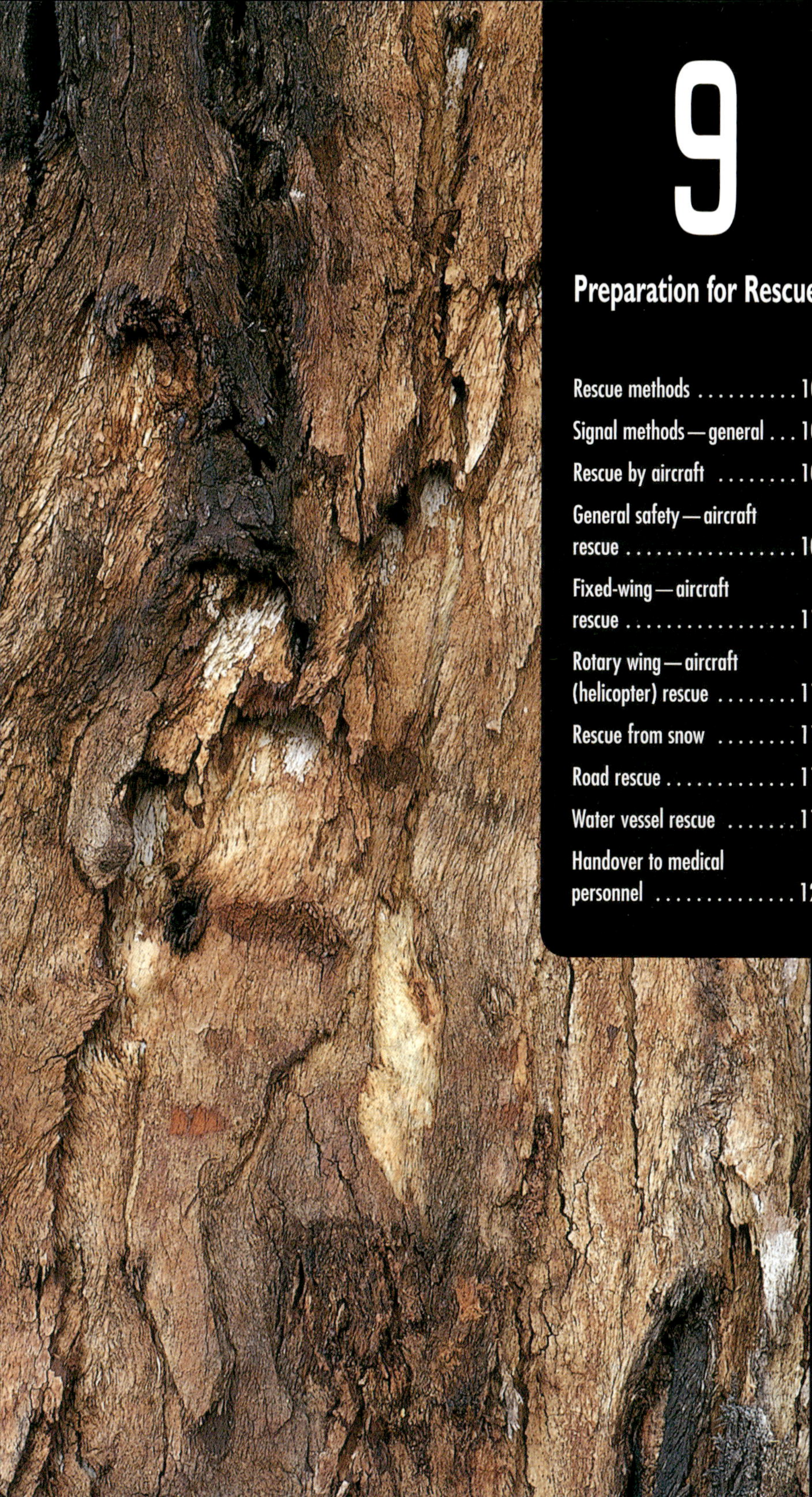

9

Preparation for Rescue

When dealing with an emergency in a remote location, preparation for rescue should commence once contact with emergency services has been made and it has been established that help is on the way. This chapter reviews steps to be taken for different types of rescue.

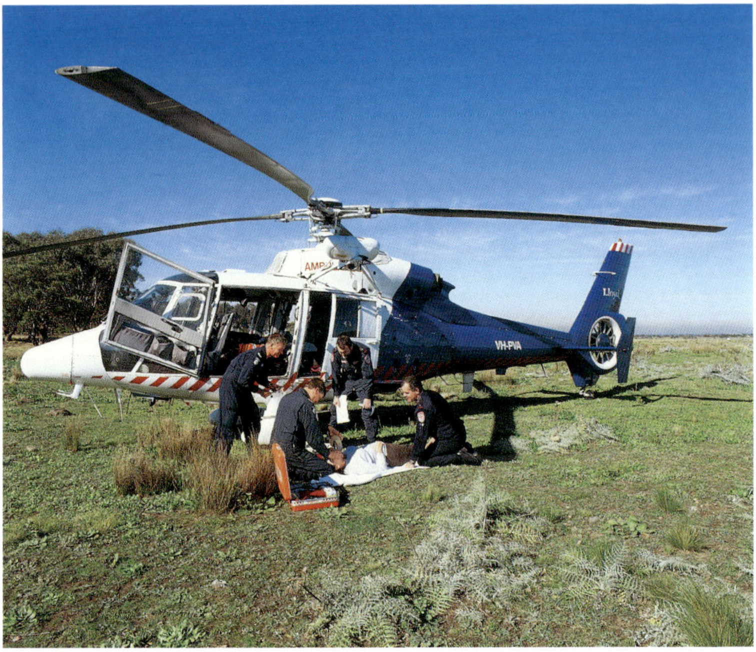

Rescue methods

A variety of rescue methods may be employed depending on the condition of the casualty and the group. These methods may include:

- fixed-wing aircraft
- rotary wing aircraft—helicopter
- foot patrols
- vehicle—road ambulance or other emergency service
- water vessel

The rescue may be carried out by military and/or civilian authorities.

Signal methods—general

Various signal methods can be used to attract attention and help guide emergency services. These methods are discussed fully in chapter five. Methods designed for a particular type of rescue may also be effective in other situations—for example the 'V' Distress Sheet *(see p. 120)*, designed for sea rescue, can also be used on land.

Distress signaling can be indicated using flares or rockets or by lighting three fires 30 m apart in a triangle or in a line.

Rescue by aircraft

Signal methods

A number of different methods can be used to communicate with aircraft. When using radio, it is important that the person on the ground managing the rescue follows the points below.

1 Remain in radio contact with the pilot prior to and during the rescue.

2 Advise the pilot of exact location of the casualty.

3 Describe the closest identifiable landmark.

Ground-to-air emergency code

If radio communication with the pilot is not possible, location aids such as ground-to-air emergency codes may be used.

These include ground markings that are dug or made with natural objects.

Ground markings must be:

- dug into sand or soft open ground, 6 x 1 m
- clearly visible from the air
- situated to provide good arcs of view from all directions

↑	Proceeding in the direction
N	No
Y	Yes
V	Require assistance
X	Unable to proceed
If in doubt use distress signal: SOS	

Alternatively, the distress signal 'SOS' can be made from rocks, greenery from trees, or branches. This is a simple method of attracting attention.

Air-to-ground emergency code

You will know if your message has been received and understood if pilot responds by:

- rocking aircraft from side to side in daylight
- flashing a green light at night

If your message has been received but NOT understood, pilot will respond by:

- flying aircraft in right-hand circles during daylight
- flashing a red light at night

General safety—aircraft rescue

1 The pilot is in sole command of the aircraft at all times. Any decision made by the pilot should be respected and not questioned even if it means aborting a rescue attempt.

2 No person may load or unload anything or enter the aircraft without the knowledge or permission of the pilot.

3 The pilot must acknowledge that you have been seen and only the pilot can give you a signal that it is safe to approach the aircraft.

4 Other than a signal fire, all fires should be extinguished if in close proximity to the landing area.

5 Smoking is not permitted at any time.

6 If possible, maintain communication with rescue authority or aircraft.

7 Casualties should be covered for protection if near landing area.

8 Ensure that you know where all team members are located.

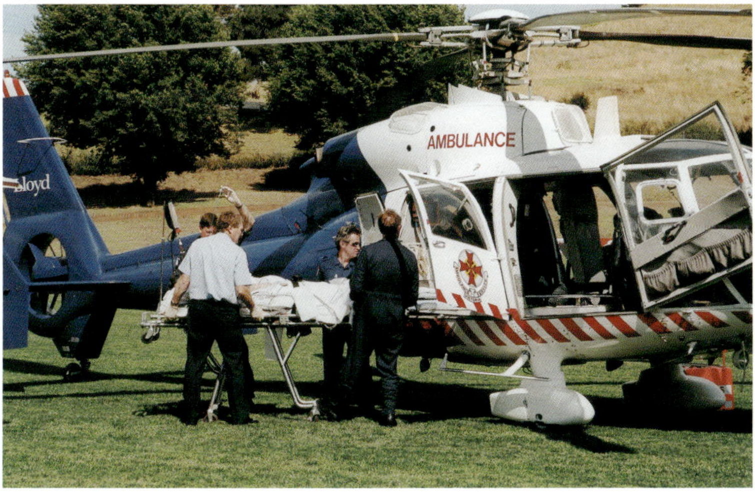

Preparing casualty for loading into aircraft

Casualties positioned close to the aircraft landing area must be covered to avoid dust and particle intrusion to wounds and eyes.

1 Carry all objects horizontally—IV containers must be turned off and placed on the stretcher.

2 Do not wear loose headwear or clothing.

3 Secure stretcher linen.

4 Secure loose materials such as bandages, straps etc. to avoid airborne debris.

5 Complete all documentation pertaining to casualty including information to be handed over to medical personnel.

6 Check adequacy of dressings, bandages and splints.

7 Reassure casualty that help will soon be arriving.

Fixed-wing aircraft rescue

If a fixed-wing aircraft, such as those of the Royal Flying Doctor Service, is used to evacuate a casualty from a bush airstrip, special guidelines need to be strictly adhered to for the safety of all concerned.

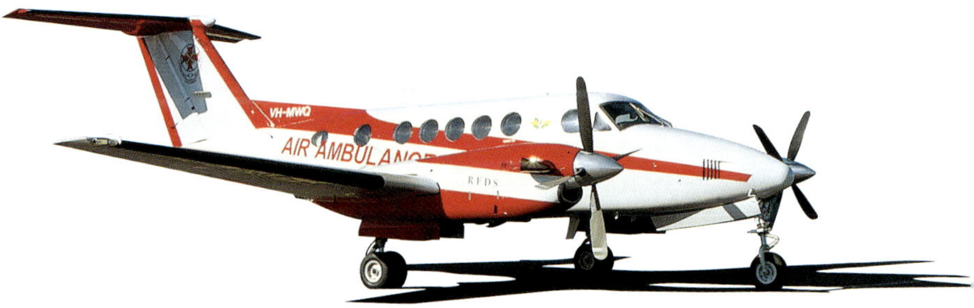

Size of runway

1 The runway should be at least 1000 m (1 km) in length—if you have a vehicle, measure length of strip using odometer/trip meter.

2 The width of the strip must be 30–40 m.

Wind direction

Aircraft always land and take off into the wind. Information about the wind direction is essential for pilots. You might need to advise the pilot of wind direction, especially if a night landing is necessary. Some bush airstrips have windsocks.

Condition of airstrip

Most bush strips are dirt and not always smooth or level.

1 Check strip for safety—make sure that there are no potholes, rocks or wandering livestock on the strip.

2 Ensure that strip is regularly slashed and cleared of bushes and undergrowth.

During the wet season, many areas of the outback become submerged—even 'all-weather' airstrips. Even after some days of hot, dry weather following heavy rain, the airstrip may remain unsafe for an aircraft to use.

If rain has fallen recently:

- drive a vehicle over the strip at no more than 10 km per hour
  - if this leaves significant wheel marks on the strip—it is unsafe for a fixed-wing aircraft

If the strip has dried out and is rough:

- drive a vehicle over it at 100 km per hour
  - any excessive bumping is an indication that the strip is not safe
  - any 'stickiness' or 'pulling' of the vehicle indicates that the strip is not safe

Lighting the airstrip

Pilots are not permitted to land on unlit bush airstrips at night, as night landings can be extremely dangerous. If landing lights are not available, the strip must be lit with emergency lighting for an incoming aircraft. The pilot must be able to see the length of the strip from the air.

Most outback stations and remote area properties that have an airstrip have commercially prepared flares for lighting the strip. Should flares be unavailable, a 5 L tin, with the top completely open, filled with rag or cotton waste soaked in kerosene, makes a usable flare when lit.

Remember: The pilot watches the line of flares, not the lit ground. It is preferable at all times to light the strip on both sides. If this is not possible due to insufficient flares or lack of time, the flares must be laid in order of priority.

Emergency lighting of airstrip

1 Lay double sets of flares at each end of the strip—flares 1 & 2 and 3 & 4 at one end of the strip, and flares 5 & 6 and 7 & 8 at the other end. Ensure that flares 2 and 3, and flares 6 and 7 are 30–40 m apart to indicate the width of the strip to the pilot.

2 Note the wind direction—an aircraft will always land into the wind.

3 Stand on the airstrip facing into the wind.

4 Place the first line of flares 90 m apart on the left side of the runway in the order of priority, noting wind direction arrows in relation to placement of flares.

5 Place the second line of flares 90 m apart on the right side of the runway in the order of priority, noting wind direction arrows in relation to placement of flares.

6 The aircraft will land from behind you as you face into the wind.

7 The left and right side on the runway must have flares evenly spaced from the beginning of the strip (behind you) to the end of the strip (in front of you).

If insufficient flares or time, lay flares in order of priority as indicated, see diagram page 113. However, it is highly recommended to have a full line of flares on each side of the runway.

Note: The following diagram shows the layout of flares as described above.

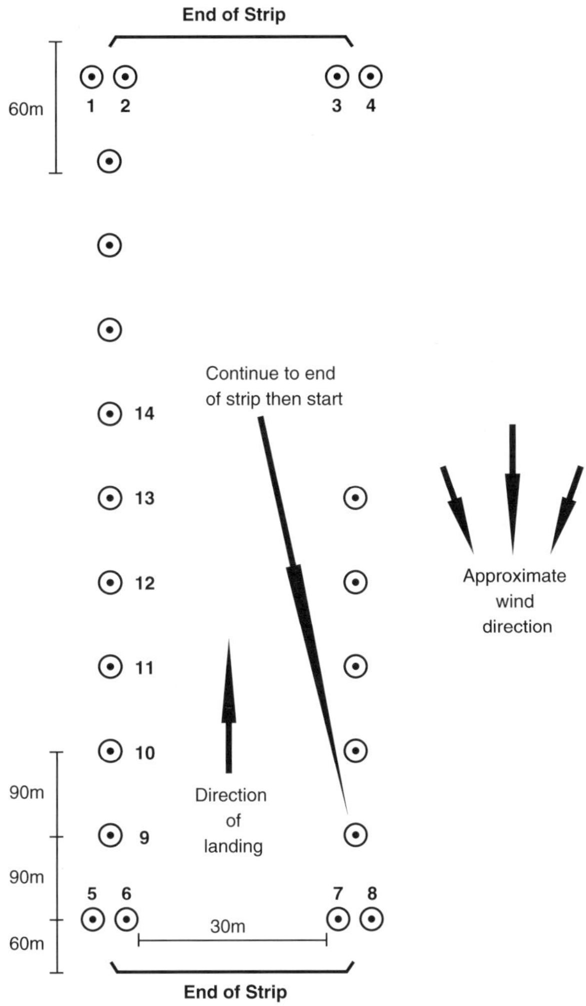

Alternative methods of lighting airstrip

RFDS aircraft will not normally land at night on strips unless lit by flares. A landing using vehicle headlights will only be undertaken in extreme medical circumstances and only at airfields familiar to the pilot.

In an emergency, improvised flares using 5 L tins can be used *(see p. 111)*.

To help the aircraft locate the landing area it is desirable to have a car or two facing into the wind, with the lights on high beam and if possible, with the front end slightly elevated on rising ground with the light beams just clear of the ground. It is suggested also that the car lights be flashed intermittently. The lights should be switched off after the aircraft has arrived in the area.

It is recommended that at all times during a night approach and landing a responsible adult stands by the radio or telephone in case communication between the pilot and the ground is required.

It is important to remember that the pilot may attempt to land a doctor even in very undesirable conditions. You must make the landing of the aircraft as safe as possible. If it is unsafe, you must make every effort to advise as accurately as possible that the strip or conditions are not safe so that the doctor can make alternative arrangements to evacuate the casualty. No matter how serious the condition of your casualty, NEVER encourage a landing if you are unsure about the safety of the airstrip.

Other safety considerations

1. **DO NOT** approach an aircraft until the propellers have stopping spinning completely.

2. Always stand well clear of the aircraft when it is taxiing, landing or taking off.

3. **DO NOT** face the rear of an aircraft that is taxiing as dust and windborne debris is driven at high velocity backwards from the propellers.

4. If a vehicle is involved, after receiving acknowledgment from the pilot to proceed, approach the plane slowly staying well clear of wings, struts and any guidewires. Park the vehicle on the side closest to rear door of aircraft and await further instruction from pilot or rescue authority.

Rotary wing aircraft (helicopter) rescue

In the event that a helicopter/rotary wing aircraft is used to evacuate the casualty, special guidelines need to be adhered to strictly for the safety of all concerned.

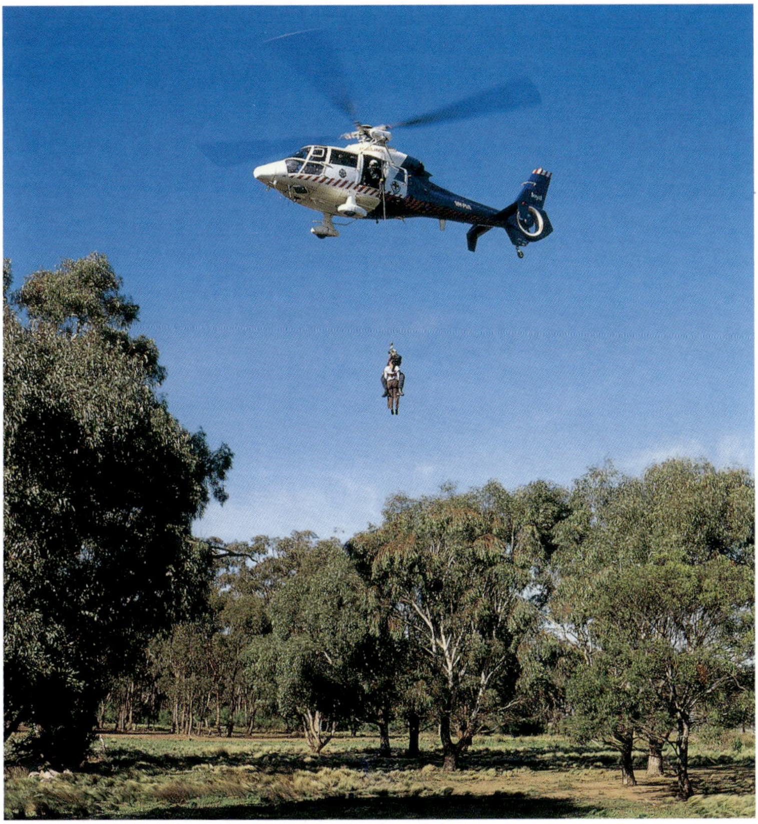

Landing space

1 A cleared space of at least 30 sq m is required.

2 The area should be as flat as possible.

3 If the area is bushy, the pilot at his/her discretion may still consider it safe to land the aircraft.

Lighting

1 If at night, check if the closest homestead will be lit.

2 Check if local lighting will be available at the actual landing site—commercial or improvised flares such as lanterns, car headlights, or kerosene-soaked rags in tins.

Other safety considerations

1 Always turn your back towards the helicopter as it is landing or taking off to avoid possible eye injuries.

2 Never approach the helicopter without the pilot giving permission by the thumbs-up signal. Wait to be guided to the aircraft by the crew.

3 Vehicles must not approach the helicopter while the rotors are turning.

4 While approaching or leaving the helicopter, anyone who is temporarily blinded by dust should immediately stand still or sit down. **DO NOT** grope or stumble around.

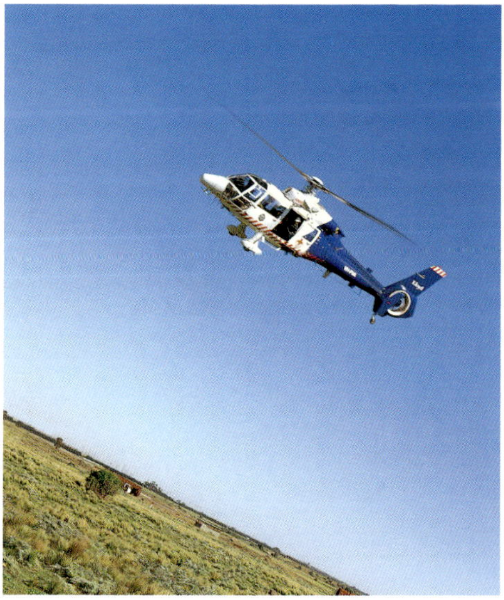

Rescue from snow

If you are injured or realise that you are lost while skiing or in snow country, seek shelter as close as possible to where you are, then remain there. In poor weather conditions, shelter behind trees or rocks and place your crossed skis above the position.

If you are equipped with camping gear, the best place to set up is on the edge of a clearing, where you can easily move out from the shelter to attract attention.

Use distress signal—three signals together regularly spaced or anything that will attract attention e.g. smoke, whistles, flashing a mirror or torch, or by distinct waving of clothing.

Decide how to best attract the rescuers. If possible wear brightly coloured clothing. A smoky fire is also a good location marker.

Wait for rescue. If you have made meeting arrangements with others, as you should, the ski patrol and other rescuers should know where to look and rescue may be close at hand.

Helicopters may be called in to rescue you in extreme circumstances. Keep well clear of the helicopter's landing area and await instructions from the pilot.

Road rescue

Rescue may be via road ambulance or other vehicle emergency service. If a person is injured or ill, if your vehicle has broken down or if you are lost, remember you are more likely to survive if you stay with your vehicle. Your vehicle will be more visible than you from the air or road.

Hopefully, you will have been able to call for help using your communications equipment. Once you have established that help is on the way, you will need to evaluate your food and equipment and manage anyone who is injured or ill. If you have a tarpaulin, sheet or similar material, attach it to the vehicle to provide shade or shelter.

Try to make visual contact—for example by laying a space blanket on the ground. This may attract rescue aircraft. Consider using an emergency beacon (EPIRB) if you have one *(see p. 58 for air rescue)*.

Water vessel rescue

Coping with emergencies and treating casualties at sea require a cool head and clear mind. The people who need to make decisions and give treatment may themselves be suffering from shock and/or injuries. The decision to seek assistance when at sea is made by the skipper or leader of the craft and is not taken lightly.

In an emergency the skipper or leader should:

1 Take control and create a calm atmosphere.

2 Ensure lifejackets are worn.

3 Choose a helmsman who can steer a safe and steady course.

4 Call for help.

5 Move casualty only if in danger.

6 Follow first aid management protocols—consider dehydration, hypothermia, hyperthermia and exhaustion.

The best way to signal that you are in trouble is by using your marine radio or some other means of two-way communication. By using two-way communications you can pass on information about your situation and answer questions so that rescuers are well-informed and can tailor the rescue to your needs.

Distress signals

If you are in a situation where you or others are threatened by grave or imminent danger and require immediate assistance then a distress call should be made. Stations that hear the distress call must immediately cease all transmissions that may interfere with distress communications. A vessel that receives a MAYDAY signal and is, without any doubt, in the vicinity should immediately acknowledge receipt. A distress call or message may be transmitted only on the authority of the master or skipper, or the person responsible for the safety of the vessel.

Distress calls consist of:

- distress signal MAYDAY spoken three times

- words THIS IS, and name and call sign of the vessel in distress spoken three times

These calls are followed by a distress message that consists of:

- distress signal MAYDAY
- name and call sign of the vessel in distress
- particulars of its position
- nature of the distress and the kind of assistance desired
- any other information which may facilitate rescue

If you are in a situation where you have concerns for a vessel's or person's safety then you should transmit an urgency signal. Such a situation might be the loss of a propeller or breakdown of engine and the urgent need for a tow.

Urgency signal consists of:

- words PAN PAN spoken three times
- station called—spoken three times (it could be all stations)
- words THIS IS
- name and call sign of the vessel, spoken three times
- URGENCY message that gives position, nature of problem and assistance required

Emergency Position Indicating Radio Beacon (EPIRB)

An EPIRB is a compact, buoyant, self-contained radio transmitter that, when activated, emits a distinctive radio signal for at least 48 hours. EPIRBs can be detected by orbiting satellites and overflying aircraft, if the aircraft are monitoring the aviation distress frequency of 121.5 MHz. Of the two types of EPIRBs generally available in Australia, the 406 MHz EPIRB can be located by the satellite system to within 5 km, while the older analogue 121.5 MHz EPIRB could be up to 20 km away from the satellite predicted position.

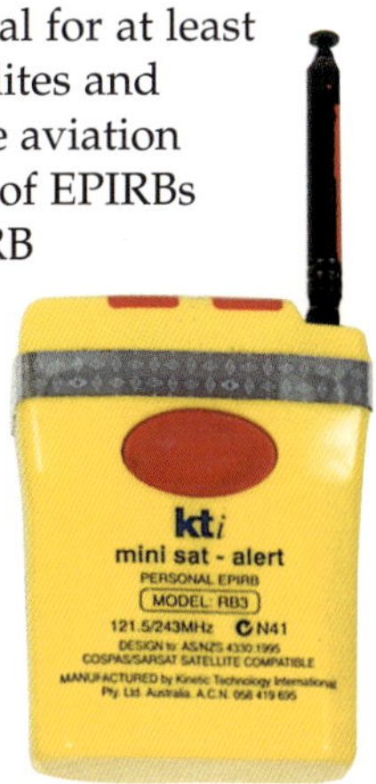

On average, an EPIRB activated off the Australian coast should be detected by the satellite system within 90 minutes. Search and rescue then commence an operation to locate and rescue you.

This may take some time so you should be prepared and carry plenty of water and food.

Because the EPIRB is not capable of transmitting speech, it should always be regarded as supplementary to and not a substitute for marine radio. Once activated, an EPIRB should not be turned off until rescue is complete or until told to do so by the search and rescue authority.

Flares and smoke

Flares and smoke can be used as signalling devices but care should be taken to ensure that there is a possibility of someone seeing the signals. Only use these signalling devices if there is a vessel or aircraft in sight or if you are close to land and would expect someone to be able to see the signal.

Signalling torch, heliograph or mirror

A torch can be used to signal aircraft and ships at night. It is directional and could be used to send a simple SOS (. . . - - - . . .) to attract attention during the day. A flashing light is more likely to be seen than steady light. The heliograph, mirror or any polished surface that will reflect sunlight are very effective methods of attracting attention. Reflected sunlight can be seen as flashes of light for many kilometres, and is an ideal means of attracting the attention of ships and aircraft.

'V' Distress Sheet

A 'V' Distress Sheet is a rectangular fluorescent orange–red sheet of material with the letter 'V' in black and makes a vessel readily visible from the air. The letter 'V' should not be less than 760 mm high and the strokes forming the 'V' not less than 130 mm wide. The sheet should not be smaller than 1.8 x 0.5 m.

Commercially made 'V' sheets are available in Australia. When used, the sheet should normally be displayed on deck or on a cabin top, or stretched over an open boat to best attract the attention of a searching aircraft. Although primarily intended to increase the chances of locating small craft from the air, the sheet may also be displayed in any manner that will attract attention and can be attached to the boat by a lanyard. If the boat capsizes, the sheet can be spread over the upturned hull.

Ship Reporting Systems

The volunteer coast guards maintain limited radio stations along the coasts where boating is popular. These stations operate on VHF and/or 27 MHz. Before putting out to sea, skippers should notify their local volunteer coast guard of their intentions. The information should include an estimated time back at the ramp or marina, where you intend to go and why. If you do not notify the local coast guard at least let a reliable friend or family member know your plans and what time you expect to return from your trip so they can inform the authorities if you do not return. Make sure they know to call the local police and that they have the number. Notify the local coast guard or your friend or family member on your return. If you are delayed make sure you make contact and update your estimate of the time you are likely to get back.

If you are making a longer voyage some coast guard stations offer a reporting system. You will be required to give the station closest to your departure place the details of your voyage and make regular daily reports of your progress. As you pass from one station to the next your details are faxed ahead ready for you to report to the next station. When you reach your destination notify the local coast guard station that you have arrived.

The Australian Maritime Safety Authority's Rescue Coordination Centre (RCC Australia) in Canberra provides a 24 -hour search and rescue service for mariners and aviators in distress in the Australian Search and Rescue Region. The police are responsible for the search and rescue of small craft and will work closely with volunteers and, if necessary, RCC Australia to effect any rescue necessary.

RCC Australia offers a reporting scheme similar to that of the volunteers known as the Small Craft Australian Ship Reporting System (SC AUSREP), a variation of the AUSREP system used for large vessels. SC AUSREP is available for smaller vessels carrying appropriate communication equipment including a licensed HF radio or Inmarsat-C and an EPIRB, and where the voyage is more than 320 km between ports.

Medical services can be sought through coast radio stations, volunteer coast guard stations and a few private marine radio stations, using the 'URGENCY' procedure if necessary. Messages should be prefixed 'RADIO MEDICAL' and state clearly the symptoms of the illness or injury and details of medical stores carried on board.

Handover to medical personnel

The handover of the casualty to medical personnel is an important aspect of your care. Information you hand over can assist in the management of the casualty in hospital. Information such as amount of body fluid lost through bleeding, burns, vomiting or diarrhoea can be essential in determining later treatment.

Checklist for handover

1 Provide all completed records pertaining to the casualty's treatment—incident report, observation chart.

2 Give a complete history of the incident.

3 Assist medical personnel further if requested.

4 Advise medical personnel of the condition of all members of your party.

Note: Medical personnel will nearly always spend time treating the casualty prior to evacuating.

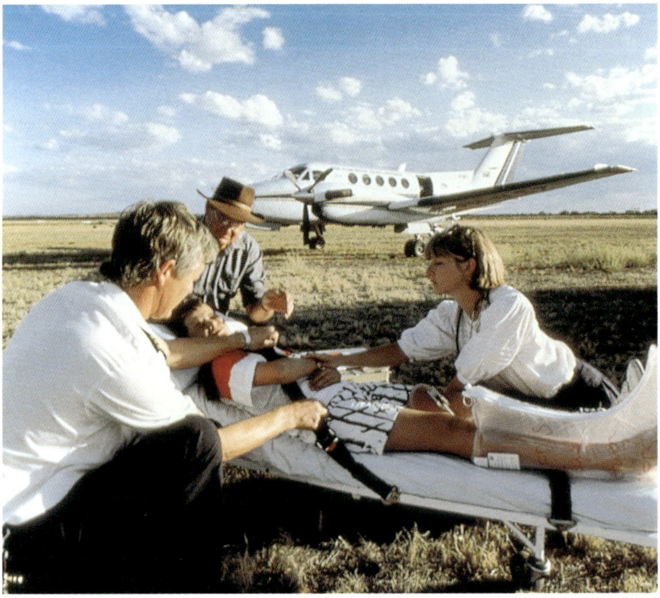

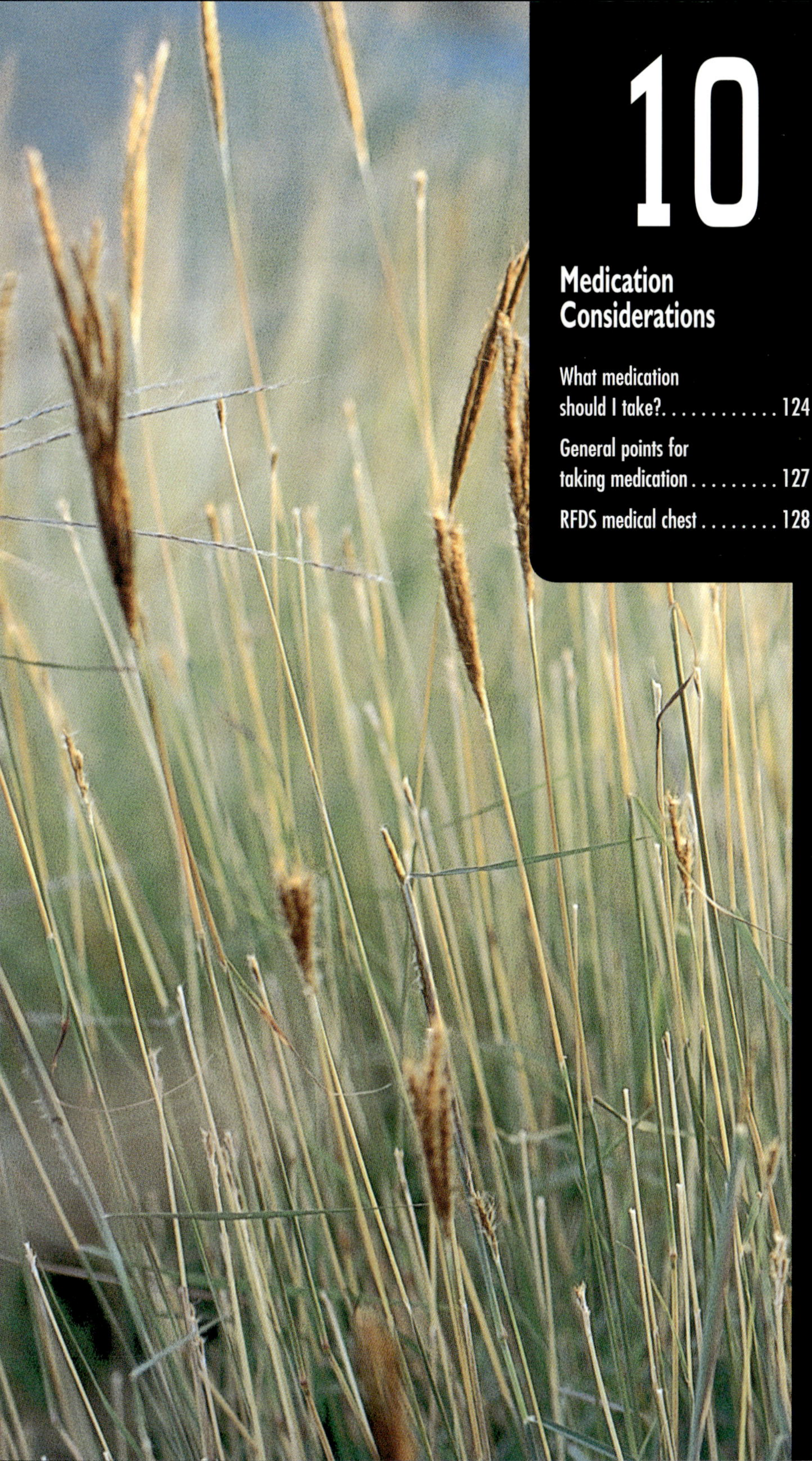

10

Medication Considerations

People who travel into remote areas, as a requirement of their job or for recreational purposes, need to consider what medication they may need to take with them.

It is generally the responsibility of people travelling in remote areas to provide their own medication. It is advisable for those who take regular medication for a condition to also carry repeat prescriptions and extra supplies.

Consult your doctor, and for overseas travel, particulary into remote locations, seek advice from the Travellers' Medical Advisory Service.

Before travelling in remote areas ensure that you are immunised against diseases found in the region. Also check with your doctor the need for a tetanus booster.

What medication should I take?

In considering what medication to take on an extended trip it is advisable that you speak with your doctor, even if the medication you wish to take can be bought 'over the counter'. A doctor will advise you of the most suitable medication for your purposes and explain the implications of its use. Your doctor may also be willing to give advice if required during your trip, provided contact can be made.

In most cases the medication we carry will remain unused. By ensuring that we have the capability to treat illnesses commonly encountered by travellers, we minimise the risk of personal discomfort, prevent the condition becoming worse and increase the likelihood of an enjoyable trip.

Note: While not viewed as drugs, sunscreen, lip balm and insect repellant are a must for most travellers.

Following are suggestions of what medication to take with you.

For pain

Analgesics—paracetamol and aspirin are two of the most commonly used drugs to relieve pain. The pain from toothache can often be temporarily relieved by one of the toothache drop preparations applied to the sore tooth with a cotton bud.

For allergies

Antihistamines—some of the older drugs could cause drowsiness but many of the newer drugs do not. Your doctor/pharmacist can advise you as to which antihistamines to use.

For severe allergies

Adrenaline—one of the increasingly talked about issues in remote area first aid is whether or not to carry medication for a severe allergic reaction. A severe allergic reaction causes swelling of the throat tissues, impeding the casualty's ability to breathe. The only medication that works in this situation is adrenaline, which must be given by injection into a muscle.

The easiest way to deal with this situation is to ask those with such allergies to provide their own medication. Both the leader and the first aider need to be aware of the allergy and the medication and be shown how and when to use it. If, as the leader or first aider on a trip, you wish to explore the possibility of carrying adrenaline, you should discuss this with a doctor. Adrenaline is available in a number of different 'packages'. The easiest method of administering adrenaline for a first aider is by EpiPen™. However this is also the most expensive.

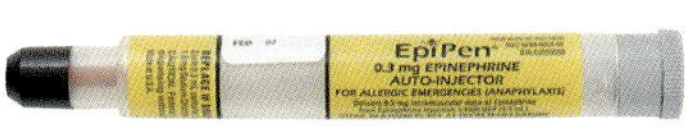

EpiPen™ (a self-injector containing adrenaline) can be used for allergic reactions

For diarrhoea

Antidiarrhoeics—can improve the level of comfort for the person with diarrhoea. However, they are not recommended for use:

- with young children
- when the person has a fever
- if blood is being passed in the faeces

For asthma

Carrying medication for asthma is generally the responsibility of the person who is likely to suffer an asthma attack. However, it is possible another member of the group may suffer an unexpected asthma attack or respiratory distress *(see p. 152)*.

Salbutamol—Ventolin, Respolin are the drugs of choice, but any of the aerosol blue/grey reliever puffers will be effective.

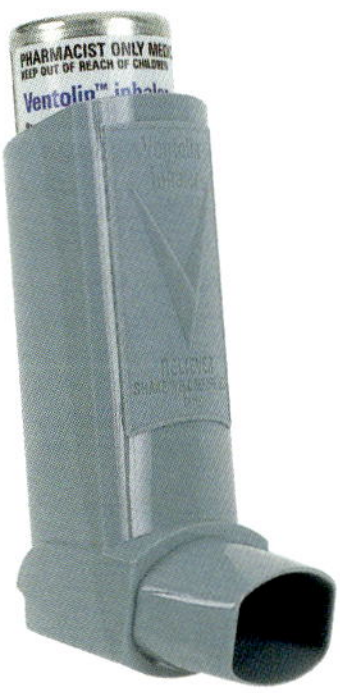

Reliever inhaler (puffer)

For infection

Antibiotics—infections, if not treated quickly, have the potential to become worse. Discuss your intended trip with your doctor who will, if appropriate, provide a prescription for antibiotics.

For tinea

Antifungals—these agents are supplied as a liquid, cream or powder and are readily available from a pharmacy.

For minor cuts and scratches

Antiseptics—e.g. Povidine Iodine; antiseptic agents help to prevent cuts and scratches from becoming infected.

General points for taking medication

Always know what you are taking and check that the correct medication has been chosen for the specific condition. Questions that should be asked of the casualty before deciding on the appropriate medication to take include:

- What would you usually take for this problem?
- Do you have any of that with you?
- Do you have any allergies to medication?
- When did you last take **any** medication?
- What was it?
- How much did you take?

Before taking or administering any medication, a number of checks need to be made:

1 Read the label to ensure it is the intended medication—check in conjunction with another person if possible.

2 Check the expiry date of the medication.

3 Follow the directions on the packaging relating to:
   - how much to take
   - how often it can be taken
   - when to take it
   - when or by whom it should not be taken.

RFDS medical chest

People who live or work in outback Australia, on remote farms or out-stations may be faced with a situation in which a member of their family or staff becomes ill or is injured. With the assistance of a Royal Flying Doctor Service (RFDS) medical chest and instructions from a doctor by radio or telephone, the ill or injured person may be treated on location. The medicine chests contain an extensive range of numbered drugs and medical supplies and are kept at remote locations across Australia, such as isolated pastoral properties, indigenous communities, out-stations, remote mining sites and lighthouses.

The medicine chest is equipped with a first aid manual, literature explaining how to describe a casualty's condition, and two charts showing the front and rear views of the human body which are mapped out to show areas of clinical importance.

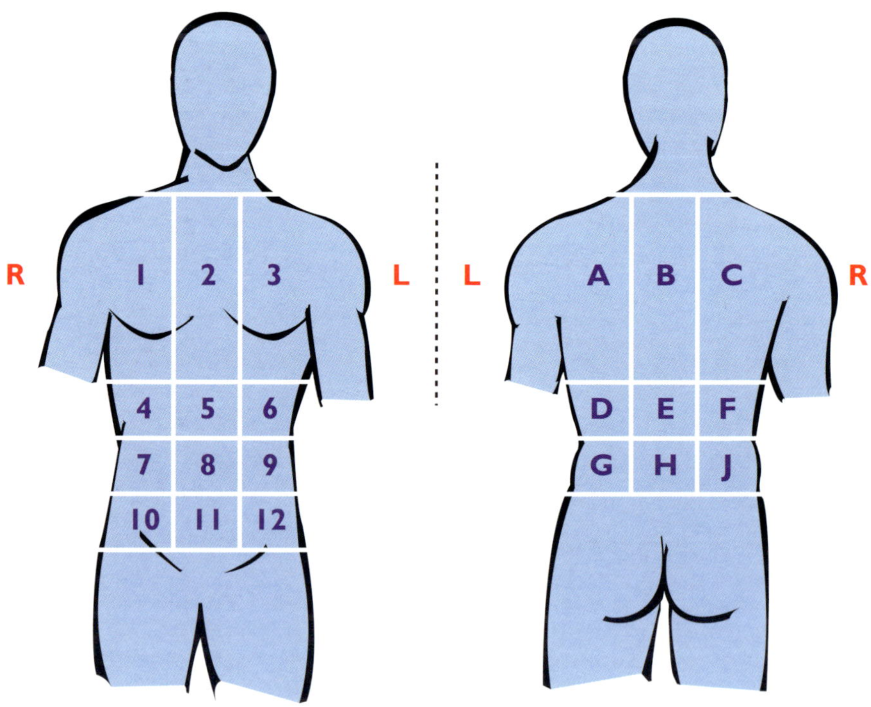

Using the RFDS medical chest

1 Call the doctor on the RFDS radio or telephone.

2 Have pen and paper ready.

3 Have the body chart handy.

4 Open the medicine chest.

5 Be ready to answer questions about the casualty's condition.

6 Listen carefully to the doctor's instructions.

7 Repeat the doctor's instructions and ask any questions if unsure.

8 Administer any treatment or medication the doctor may order.

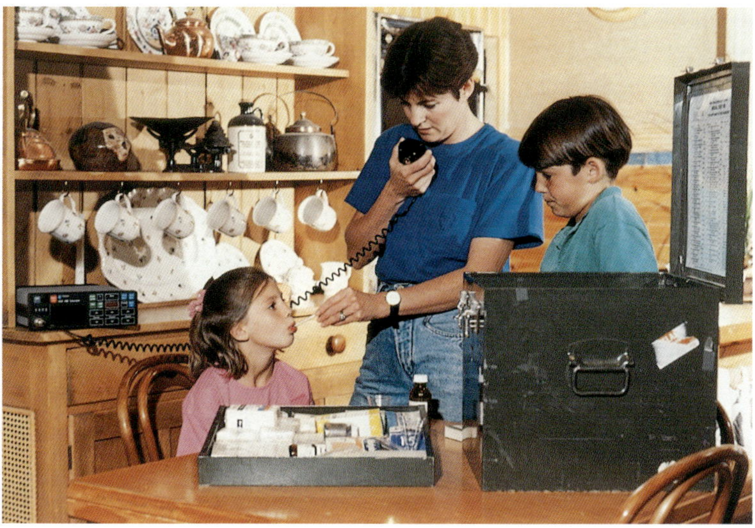

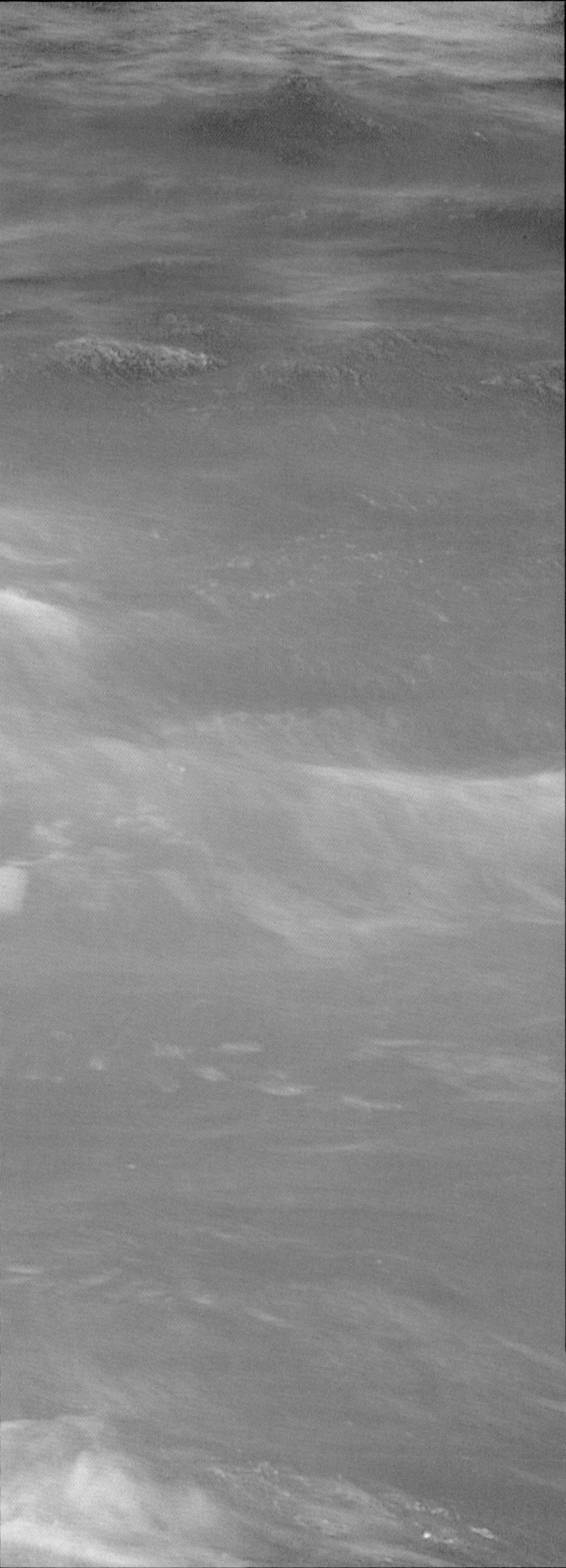

11

Emergency First Aid

A quick guide to first aid in a remote area

This chapter provides easy-to-follow steps for first aid management in a remote area. However, it is recommended that first aid skills are best acquired by completing a first aid course with a Registered Training Organisation such as St John Ambulance Australia.

The St John DRABC Action Plan is vital to the first aider in assessing whether the casualty has any life-threatening illnesses or injuries and if any immediate first aid is necessary.

DRABC

D check for DANGER

- to you
- to others
- to casualty

R check RESPONSE

- is casualty conscious?
- is casualty unconscious?

A check AIRWAY

- is airway clear of objects?
- is airway open?

B check for BREATHING

- is chest rising and falling?
- can you hear casualty's breathing?
- can you feel the breath on your cheek?

C check for CIRCULATION

- can you feel a pulse?
- can you see any obvious signs of life?

DRABC in action

**ASSESS SCENE FOR DANGER—
ENSURE IT IS SAFE**

ASSESS CASUALTY'S RESPONSE

RESPONSIVE (conscious)

Make comfortable.

Manage injury/illness.

Monitor level of consciousness, breathing, pulse, skin colour.

UNRESPONSIVE (unconscious or semi-conscious)

Place on side in recovery position.

ASSESS CASUALTY'S AIRWAY

Clear and open airway.

Tilt head back and slightly down.

Call 000 for ambulance or emergency services on mobile phones or radio

ASSESS CASUALTY'S BREATHING

BREATHING	NOT BREATHING
Leave on side.	Place on back.
Manage bleeding.	**START EAR**
Manage injury/illness.	Give 2 effective breaths.
Monitor level of consciousness, breathing, pulse, skin colour.	

ASSESS CASUALTY'S CIRCULATION (PULSE)

PULSE	NO PULSE
If **not** breathing **CONTINUE EAR.**	**START CPR.**

Adult/child over 9 yrs

1 breath every 4 seconds (15 breaths per minute)	15 compressions & 2 breaths (4 cycles per minute)

Child/baby to 8 yrs

1 breath every 3 seconds (20 breaths per minute)	5 compressions & 1 breath (12 cycles per minute)

Check pulse and breathing about every minute.

Two person CPR for an adult or child—5 compressions to 1 breath in 5 seconds (12 cycles per minute)

Note: See page 144 for further resuscitation considerations in a remote area.

Recovery Position

Adult/Child (from age 1)

1 Position casualty's legs:

- kneel beside casualty
- straighten casualty's limbs
- lift nearer leg at knee so it is fully bent upwards.

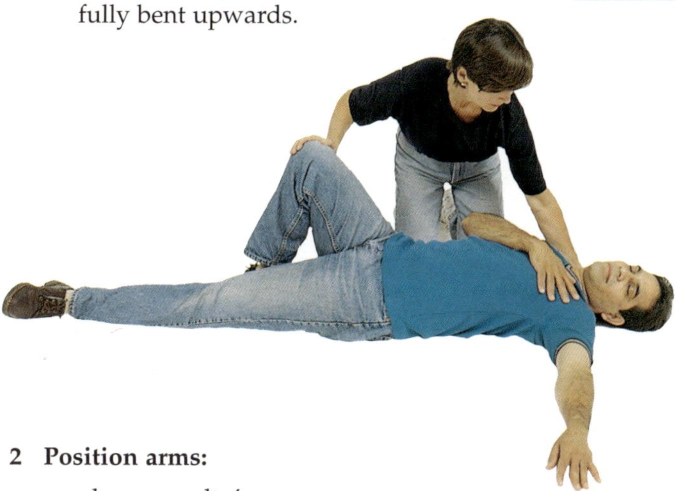

2 Position arms:

- place casualty's nearer arm across chest
- place farther arm at right angles to body.

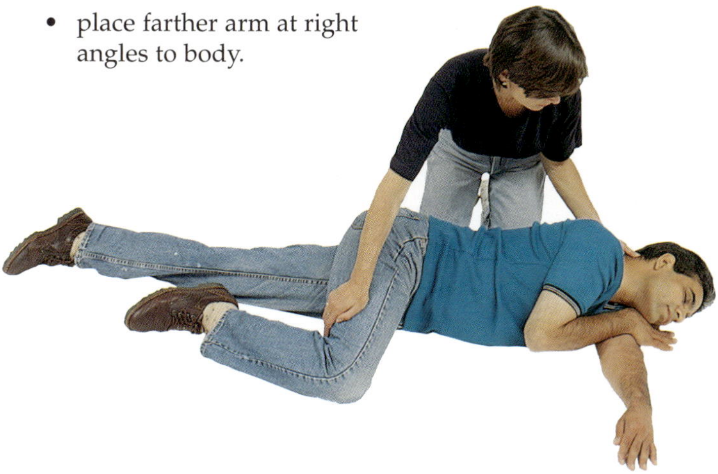

WARNING

If casualty has head or neck injuries:

Ensure head and neck are supported at all times.

DO NOT allow rotation between head and spine.

DO NOT tilt head back if neck injury suspected.

3 Roll casualty into position:

- roll casualty away from you onto side
- keep leg at right angles, with knee touching ground to prevent casualty rolling onto face.

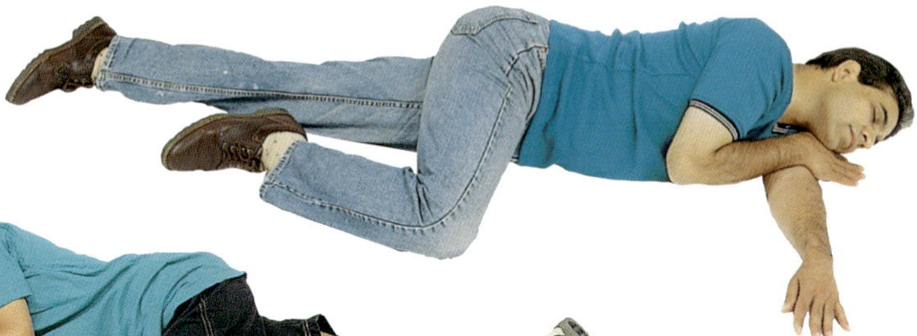

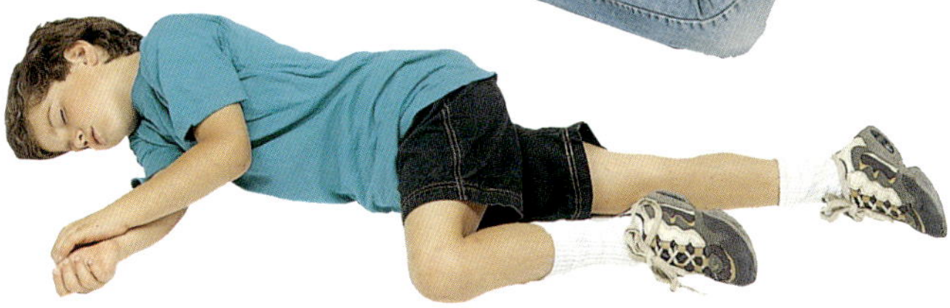

Recovery position for a child

4 Ensure airway is open.

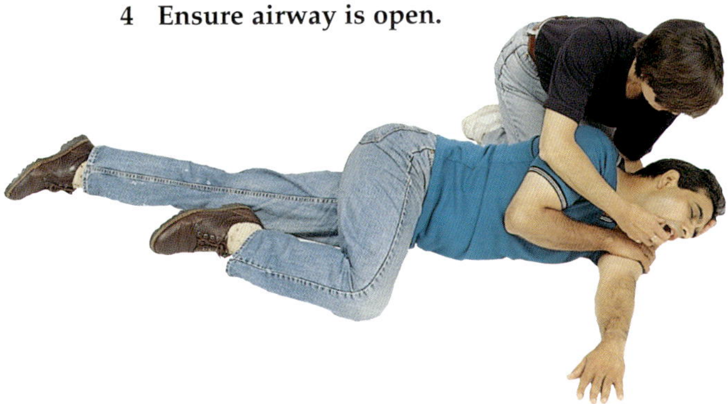

Infant recovery position

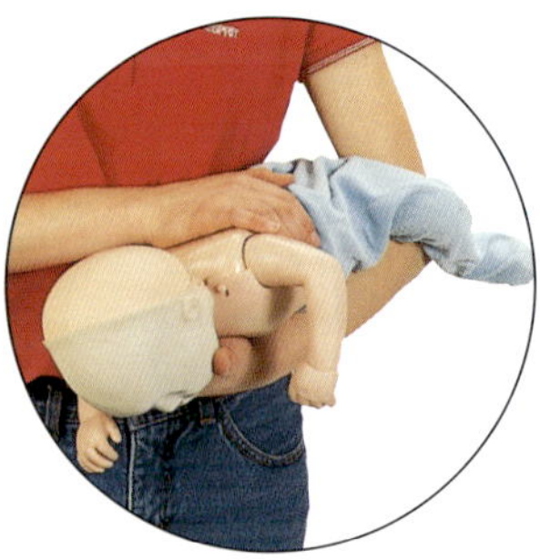

Infant (under 1)

- lay infant face down on an adult's forearm
- support head with hand
- check infant does not choke on tongue or inhale vomit

Expired Air Resuscitation (EAR)

Adult

1 Clear airway:

- place casualty in recovery position
- lift chin and open mouth
- use finger to remove any obvious obstruction
- tilt head back gently
- check breathing for up to 10 seconds.

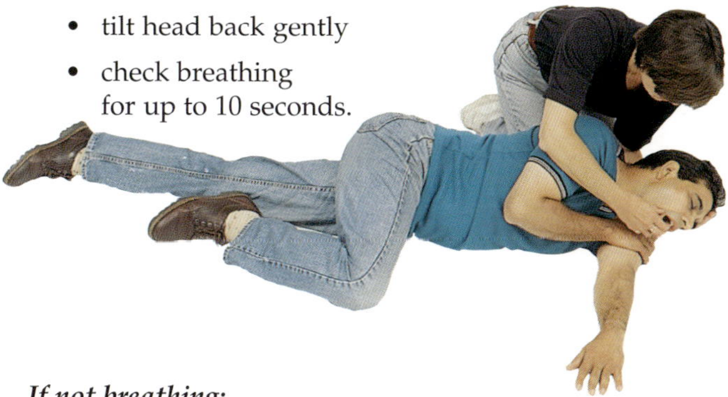

If not breathing:

2 Open airway:

- turn casualty onto back
- gently tilt head back
- pinch nose closed (use thumb and index finger)
- open mouth and maintain chin lift.

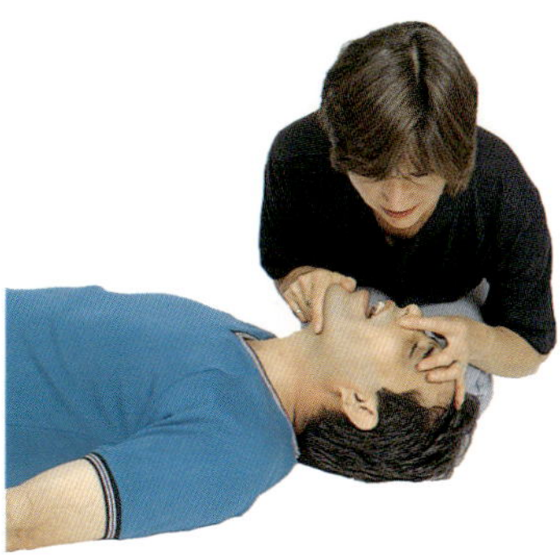

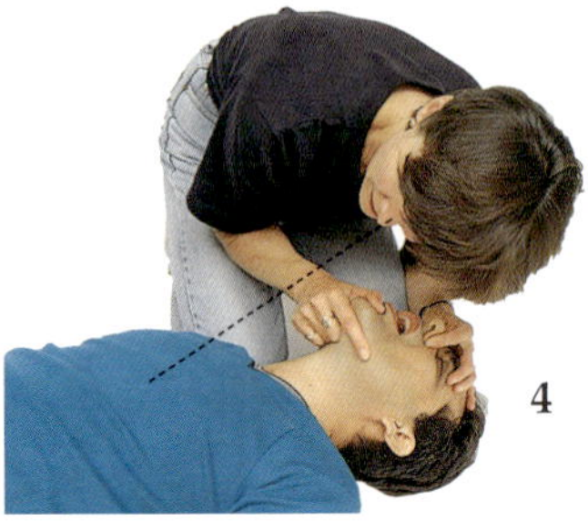

3 **Give EAR:**

- take a full breath and blow steadily into mouth for 1.5–2 seconds
- watch for chest to rise—take mouth away and watch for chest to fall
- take another breath and repeat sequence, to give two effective breaths.

4 **Check for pulse:**

- check pulse at neck or wrist
- if pulse absent, commence CPR *(see p. 141)*
- if pulse present, continue EAR at 15 breaths per minute
- recheck pulse and look for other signs of recovery about every minute.

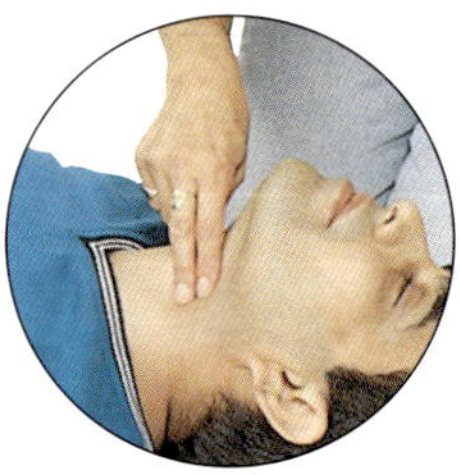

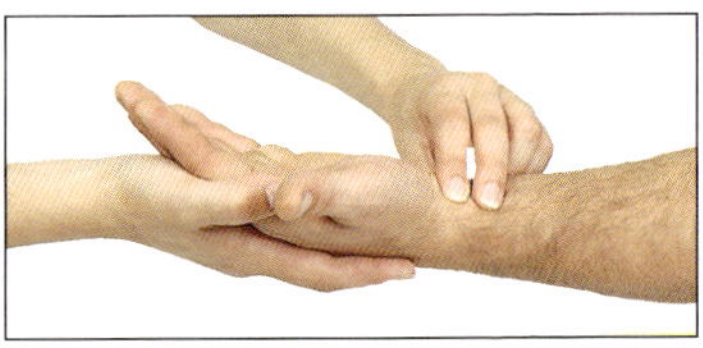

5 **Place in recovery position if breathing returns.**

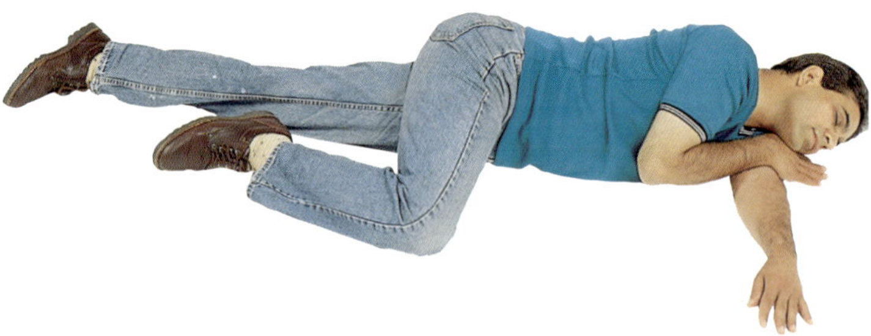

NOTE

Older child (from age 9)—use adult EAR and CPR resuscitation techniques.

Infant (under 1 year)
Child (aged 1–8)

1 **Clear airway:**

- place infant/child in recovery position
- lift chin and open mouth

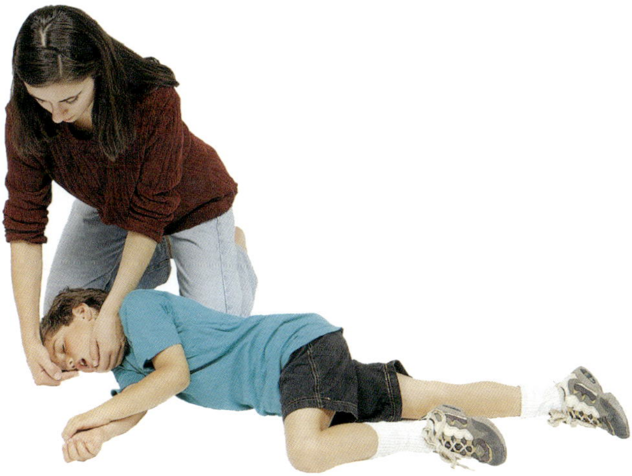

- use finger to remove any obvious obstruction
- tilt head back very gently
- check breathing for up to 10 seconds.

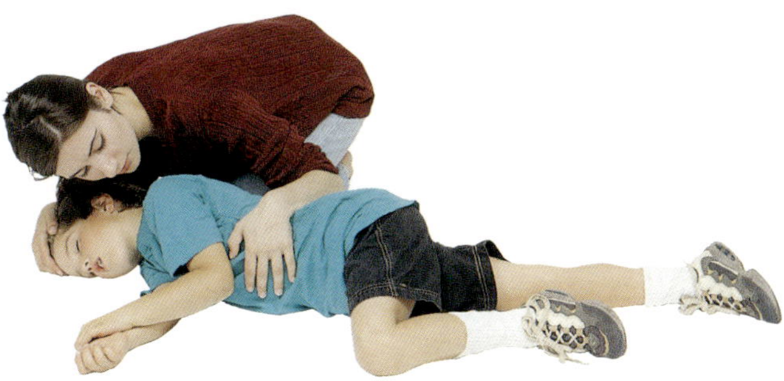

If not breathing:

2 **Open airway:**

- turn casualty onto back
- tilt head back slightly
- open mouth and lift chin.

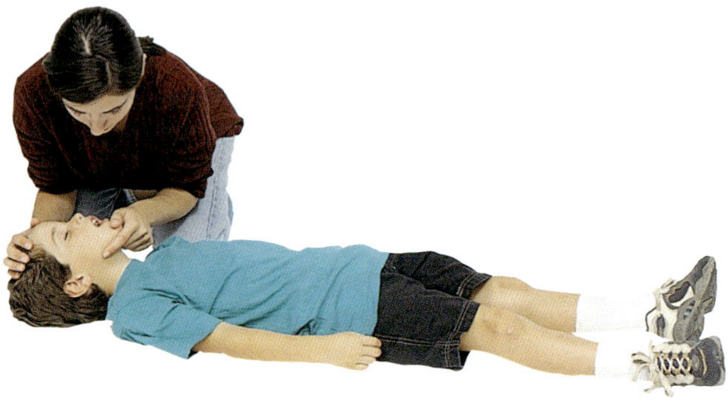

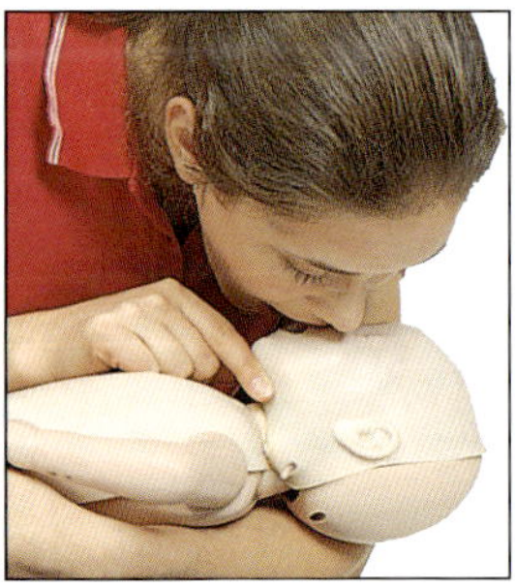

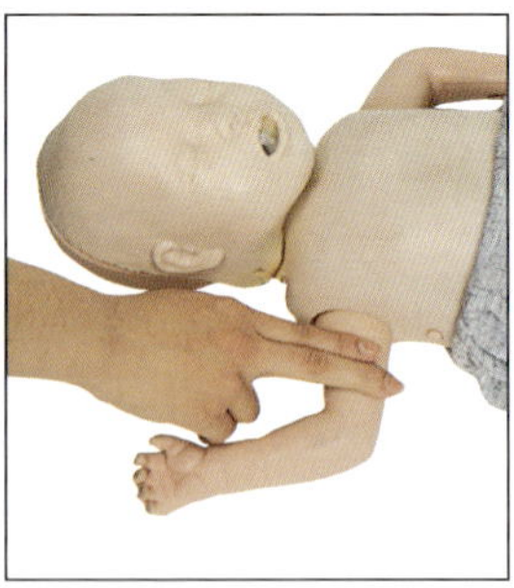

3 **Give EAR:**

- cover mouth and nose with your mouth
- give two gentle breaths/puffs into child's/infant's mouth and nose
- check pulse—infant on inside upper arm, child at neck or wrist
- if pulse absent, commence CPR *(see p. 143)*
- if pulse present, continue EAR at 20 breaths per minute
- recheck pulse and look for other signs of recovery about every minute.

4 **Place in recovery position if breathing returns.**

Cardiopulmonary Resuscitation (CPR)

NOTE

CPR combines chest compressions with Expired Air Resuscitation (EAR).

CPR is given when casualty is not breathing and has no pulse.

Adult

1 Position hands for CPR:

- place casualty on back
- find groove at neck between collarbones
- find lower end of breastbone by running finger along last rib to centre of body
- extend thumb of each hand equal distances to meet in middle of breastbone

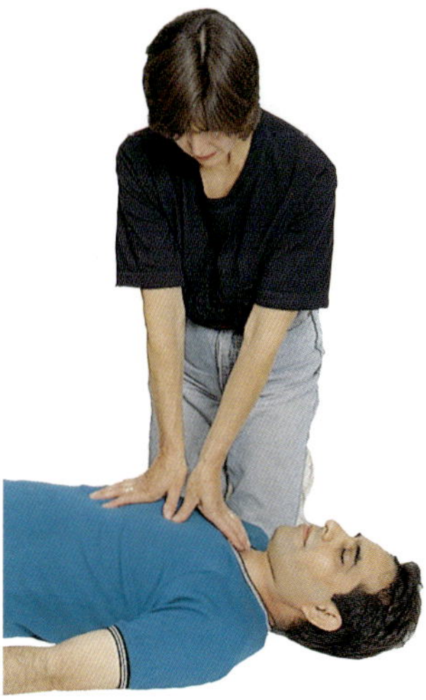

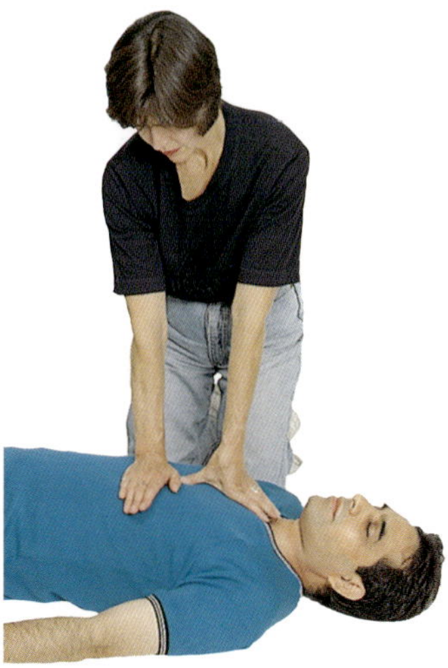

- keep thumb of one hand in position and place heel of other hand below it
- place heel of other hand on top of first and interlock fingers of both hands.

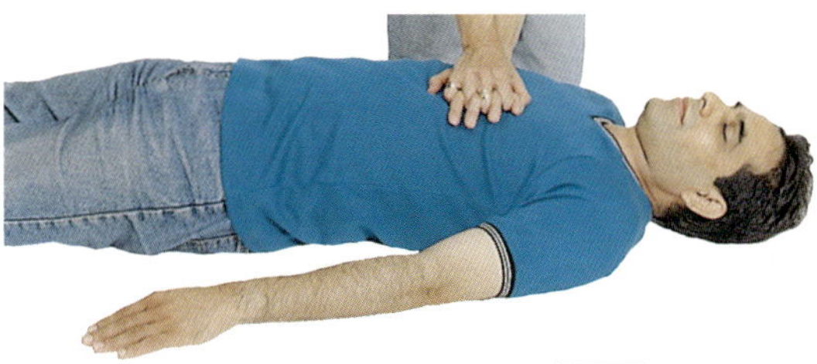

2 Commence chest compressions:

- position yourself vertically above casualty's chest
- with your arms straight, press down on breastbone to depress it about 4–5 cms
- release pressure.

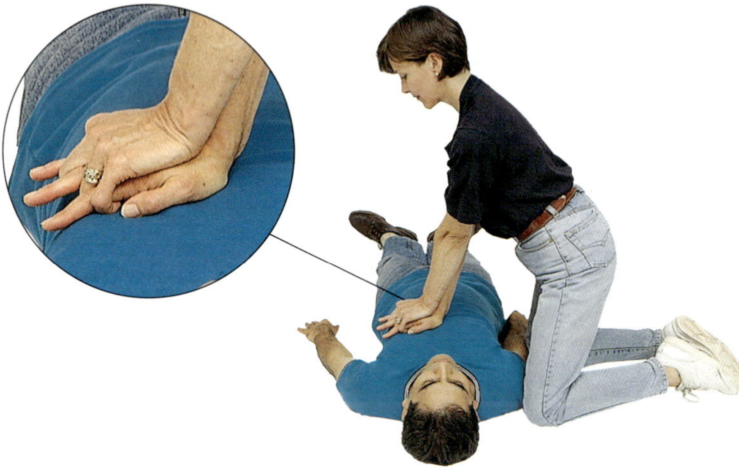

3 Continue CPR:

- complete 15 compressions
- give two effective breaths (EAR)
- continue compressions and breaths in ratio of 15:2 at a rate of 4 cycles per minute
- check pulse about every minute.

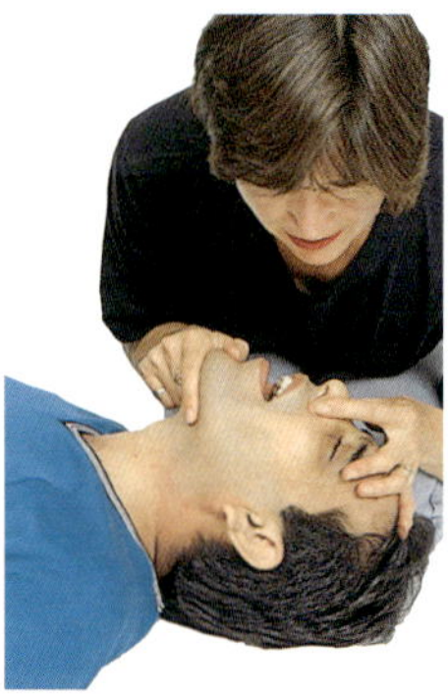

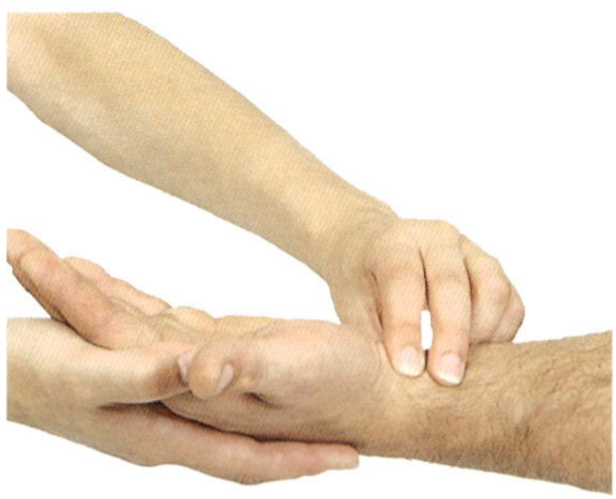

Child (aged 1–8)

- use heel of one hand over lower half of breastbone to give chest compressions
- compress chest approximately 1/3 depth of chest
- give 5 chest compressions in 3 seconds
- give 1 effective breath (EAR)
- continue compressions and breaths in ratio of 5:1 at a rate of 12 cycles per minute
- check pulse about every minute

NOTE

CPR combines chest compressions with Expired Air Resuscitation (EAR).

CPR is given when casualty is not breathing and has no pulse.

For newborn baby, chest compressions should not be attempted by anyone untrained in neonatal resuscitation.

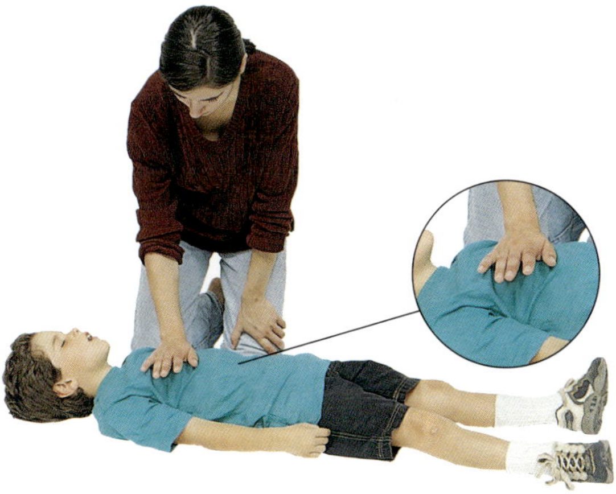

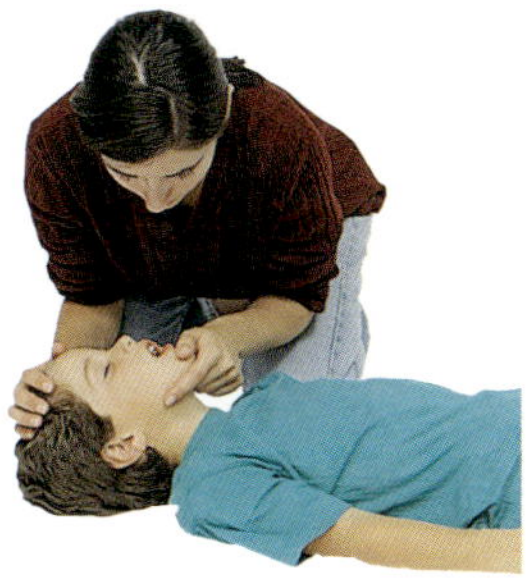

Infant (under 1 year)

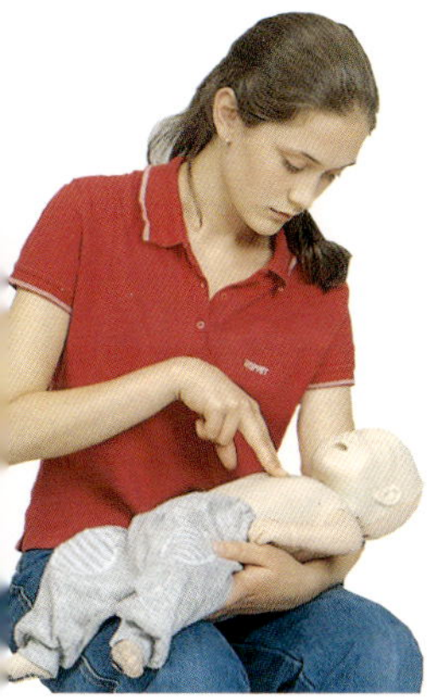

- place tips of 2 fingers (index and middle) on lower half of breastbone
- compress chest approximately 1/3 depth of chest
- give 5 chest compressions in 3 seconds
- give 1 effective breath
- continue compressions and breaths in ratio of 5:1 at a rate of 12 cycles per minute
- check pulse about every minute

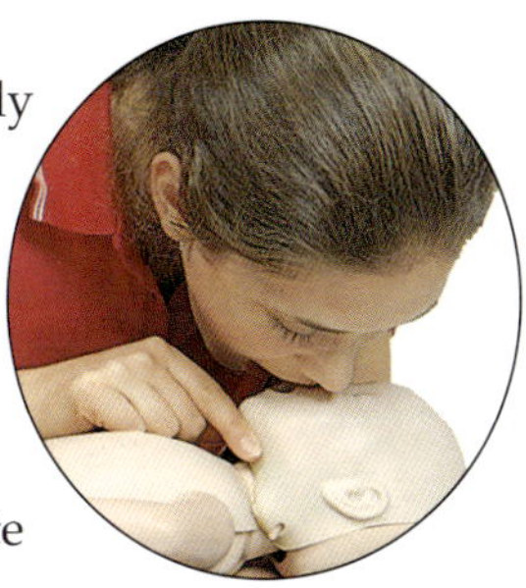

Resuscitation considerations

How long do you continue?

In an urban situation, CPR should continue until an ambulance arrives.

In a remote situation, the decision of how long you continue is more difficult. As a guide, in the absence of any response continue CPR as long as you are able or until you are advised by a medical authority to cease efforts. After 30–40 minutes without a response, further CPR is unlikely to succeed.

Consider the emotional needs of yourself and the rest of the party if CPR does not succeed, or needs to be abandoned.

CPR and hypothermia

The pulse of a seriously hypothermic casualty is often very difficult to find. In cases where severe hypothermia is suspected, take up to 45 seconds to check for pulse.

An excessively low body temperature increases the chance of survival. Therefore, if casualty being resuscitated is hypothermic, CPR should be continued uninterrupted until arrival at hospital—taking the remoteness of the situation into consideration.

Note: If the time to reach a hospital is excessive, it may be better to assume that the casualty has a weak but undetectable pulse (i.e. the person is in a 'metabolic icebox') and simply insulate casualty from further heat loss (do not rewarm and do not start CPR). If there is a weak, slow pulse, attempts at chest compressions may convert the slowly beating heart to ventricular fibrillation.

Choking

Adult

Partial blockage:

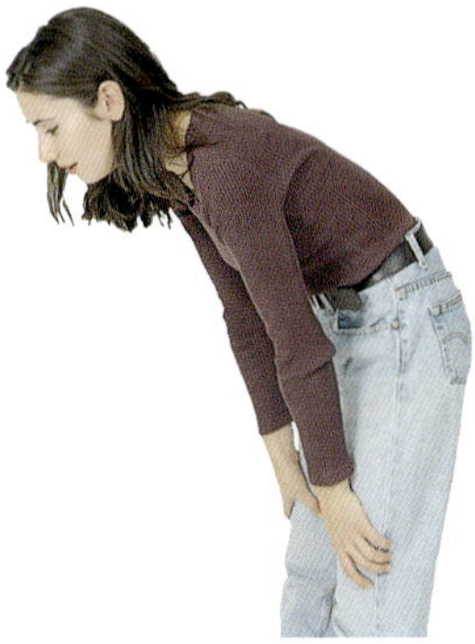

- encourage casualty to relax, breathe deeply and cough
- if unsuccessful, give 4 sharp blows between shoulderblades
- if still unsuccessful, place casualty on side on floor or ground:

  Call Emergency Services

Total blockage:

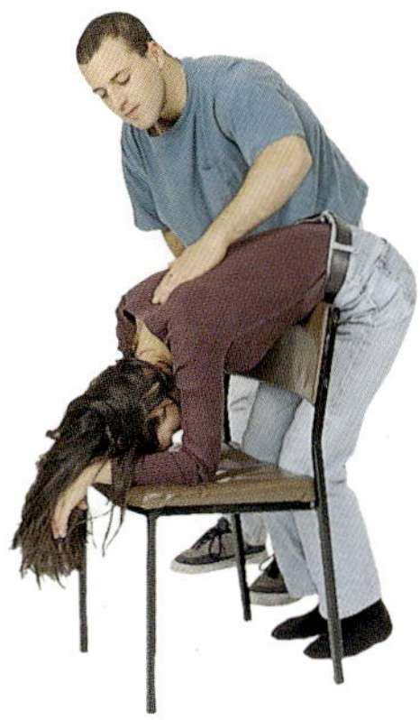

- lie casualty on side on floor or ground
- give 4 sharp blows between shoulderblades
- if unsuccessful, give 4 quick downward lateral chest thrusts (place your hands on side of chest, below casualty's armpit)
- if still unsuccessful:

  Call Emergency Services

- repeat steps until help arrives or blockage clears
- follow DRABC

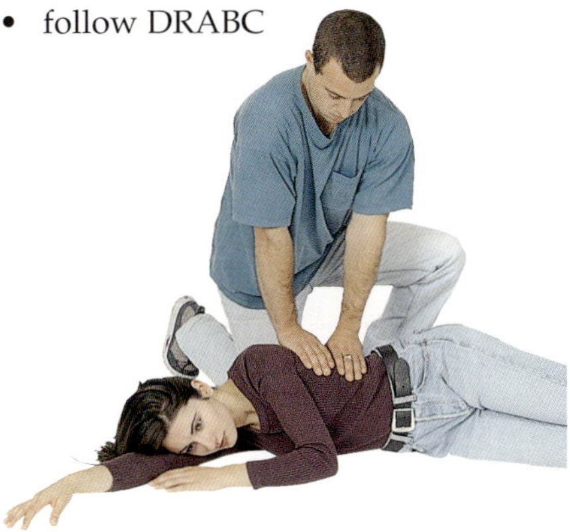

NOTE

Older child (from age 9) —manage as for adult.

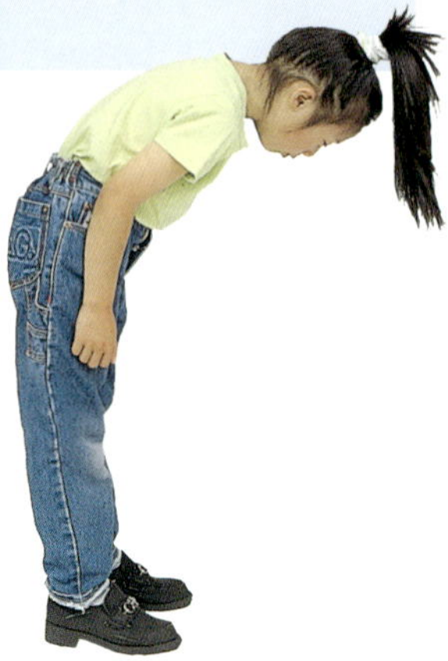

Child (1–8 years)

Partial blockage:

- ask child to try to cough up obstruction
- if unsuccessful, place child with head low and face down
- give 4 sharp blows between the shoulderblades

Total blockage:

- place child face down on the floor, ground or across your lap
- give 4 sharp blows between shoulderblades
- if not breathing, give up to 4 quick, squeezing lateral chest thrusts on both sides simultaneously (place your hands below child's armpits)
- if still unsuccessful:

  Call Emergency Services
- repeat above steps until help arrives or blockage clears
- if not breathing, follow DRABC

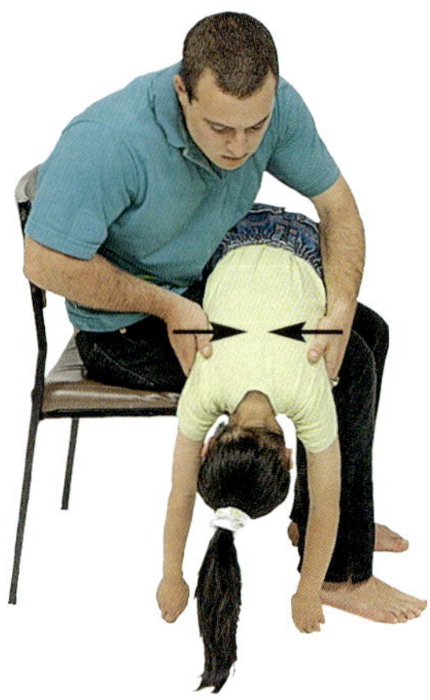

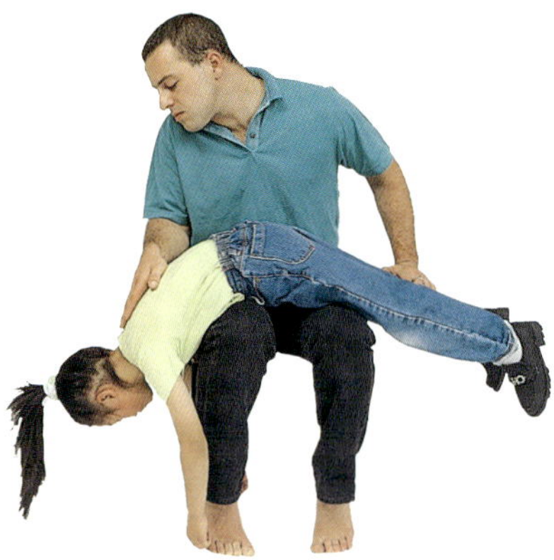

Infant (to 1 year)

Partial blockage:

- lie infant face down on your forearm with head low
- support infant's head and shoulders on your hand
- give 4 sharp slaps between shoulders
- check in infant's mouth and remove any obstruction that has come loose
- if still unsuccessful:

  Call Emergency Services

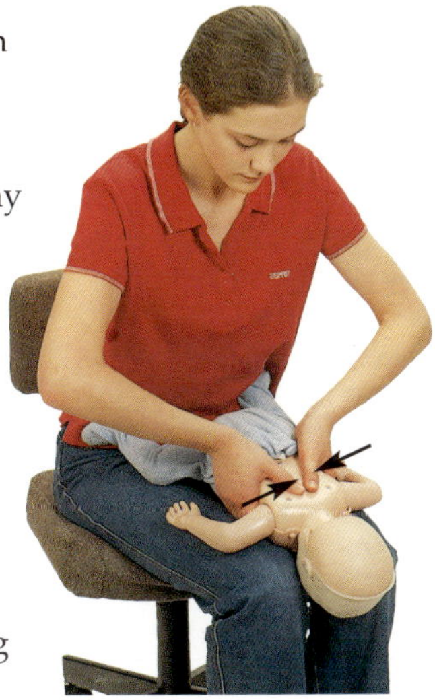

Total blockage:

- place infant face down on your lap
- give 4 sharp slaps between shoulders and check for signs of breathing
- if not breathing, give 4 quick squeezing lateral chest thrusts on both sides simultaneously (place your hands below infant's armpits)
- check in infant's mouth and remove any obstruction that has come loose
- if still unsuccessful:

  Call Emergency Services

- repeat above steps until help arrives or blockage clears
- follow DRABC

WARNING

Shock is progressive—unless recognised and treated early, it could become life-threatening.

Signs & symptoms

- weak, rapid pulse
- cooling or cold, clammy skin
- rapid breathing

Causes

- blood loss, burns
- severe diarrhoea/vomiting
- following a heart attack

Enhanced by

- pain, infection
- broken bones, poisoning

Shock

1 **Lie casualty down with head flat:**
- insulate casualty from ground
- reassure casualty.

2 **Assess casualty:**
- follow DRABC
- assess for injuries
- if possible manage cause e.g. stop bleeding.

3 ***Call Emergency Services.***

4 **Manage any other injuries:**
- if no indication of neck injury or broken leg—raise legs above level of chest
- manage wounds or burns
- immobilise fractures *(see p. 165)*
- loosen tight clothing
- cover and keep casualty comfortably warm.

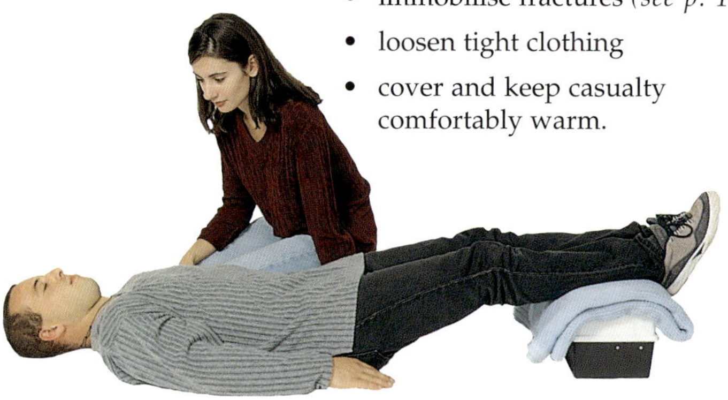

5 **Normally do not give anything to eat or drink, but if help is not expected for many hours, give small frequent sips of water.**

6 **Place in recovery position if:**
- casualty has difficulty breathing
- is likely to vomit
- becomes unconscious.

Severe bleeding

1 **Apply pressure to the wound:**

- remove or cut casualty's clothing to expose wound
- apply direct pressure over wound
- cover wound with sterile or clean dressing
- apply a pad.

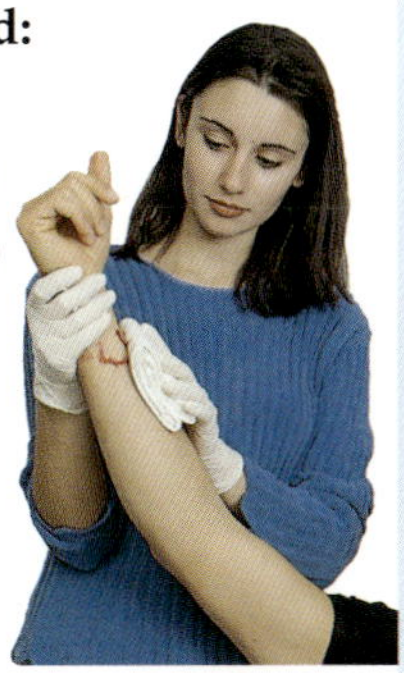

2 **Raise and support injured part:**

- lie casualty down
- raise injured part above level of heart
- handle gently if you suspect a fracture.

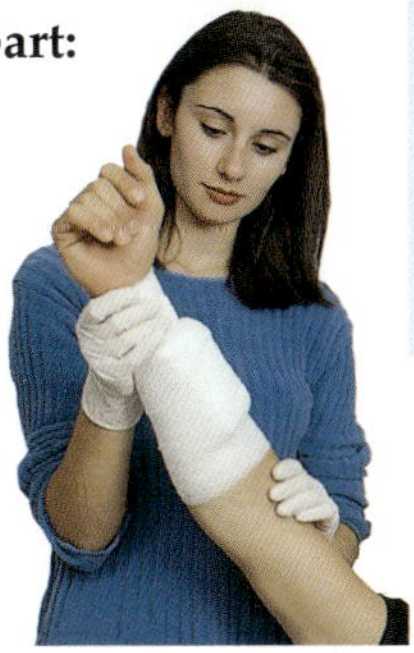

3 **Bandage wound:**

- bandage pad firmly in place
- apply another dressing or pad if bleeding continues.

4 **Check circulation below wound.**

5 ***Call Emergency Services if bleeding persists.***

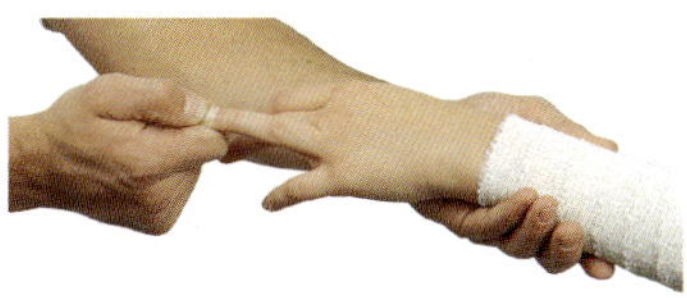

6 **Treat for shock:**

- *(see p. 148)*

WARNING

DO NOT apply a tourniquet.

If bleeding from a limb does not stop, apply pressure with hand to pressure point.

If embedded object in wound, apply pressure either side of wound and place pad around it before bandaging.

If casualty becomes unconscious, follow DRABC *(see p. 132)*

If available wear gloves or wash hands. Dispose of contaminated items—double bag and carry out as rubbish.

Wounds

When managing wounds in remote areas consider:

- is the wound bleeding heavily?
- is it a minor or major wound?
- can the wound be cleaned effectively?
- is the wound a serious risk?

The aim is to stop bleeding quickly. Severe uncontrolled bleeding may cause shock or death. Wound management is secondary to controlling bleeding *(see p. 149)*. To reduce infection in scratches or abrasions, or in small shallow cuts (less than 2 cm long and without exposed fat tissue), follow the steps below.

1 **Take precautions:**

- wash your hands
- clean wound thoroughly—with fresh clear water or saline solution
- if wound cannot be thoroughly cleaned, apply an antiseptic, e.g. povidine iodine

2 **Dress the wound:**

- apply a sterile or clean dry dressing attach firmly, e.g. with tape or bandage
- wash your hands

3 ***Call Emergency Services if wound is:***

- large, deep and penetrating
- painful, red, swollen, possibly discharging, or if casualty is feeling unwell or unable to rest properly
- small, but with serious consequences, e.g. blister that becomes infected preventing casualty from walking.

WARNING

DO NOT disturb pads that are controlling bleeding. Removing a pad to inspect a wound may cause further bleeding and/or infection.

Wounds can become infected, particularly in hot, humid conditions, within hours. Frequent handling may also increase the risk of infection *(see p. 18)*.

Signs & symptoms of infection

- pain, swelling
- redness around the wound
- discharge—may have an offensive odour
- casualty feels unwell, headache, loss of energy, chills and fever

Note

Washing discharge from wound, applying antiseptic and keeping the wound covered may reduce infection and the need for medical aid. If antibiotics are available, and have been prescribed by a doctor, they should be taken as soon as infection is noticed, e.g. pain and redness.

Chest pain or discomfort

WARNING: Treat situation as life-threatening.

1 **Advise casualty to rest:**
- advise casualty to stop any activity, and sit or lie down and rest
- protect casualty from the environment—heat, cold and wind.

2 **Casualty to take medication:**
- if casualty has medication for angina, assist casualty in taking it.

3 **Seek urgent medical attention:**
- if unconscious, follow DRABC:

Call Emergency Services immediately.

4 **Give aspirin:**
- give 300 mg (one tablet) of aspirin in water if medical aid will be delayed more than 30 minutes
- **DO NOT** give aspirin to those allergic to it, to asthmatics or those on anti-coagulant medication (e.g. warfarin).

5 **Monitor vital signs:**
- monitor pulse, breathing, consciousness, skin colour
- if the casualty looks sick, then the casualty is sick
- be prepared to give CPR *(see p. 141)*.

SIGNS & SYMPTOMS

Angina
- pain or discomfort in centre of chest
- pain radiating to neck and arms
- onset with exercise or emotional stress
- pain relieved by rest or medication

Heart attack
Signs and symptoms similar to angina, and may include:
- severe, vice-like chest pain
- anxiety/confusion
- shortness of breath
- nausea/vomiting
- irregular pulse
- sometimes immediate collapse

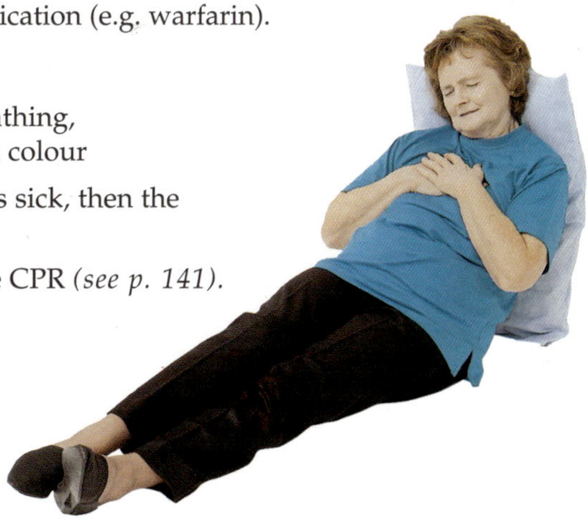

WARNING

If someone is having difficulty breathing, but has not previously had an asthma attack, and is conscious—follow the asthma attack management steps according to the severity of the attack.

Where permitted under local legislation/regulations and if necessary:

Use another person's reliever inhaler or use one from a first aid kit to assist a casualty with a severe asthma attack.

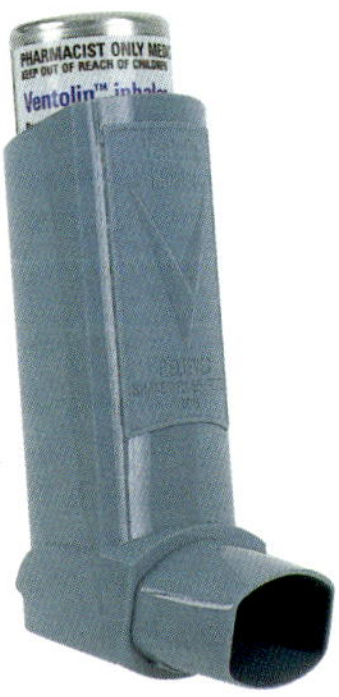

Reliever inhaler (puffer)

Asthma attack

If casualty unconscious:

- follow DRABC
- *Call Emergency Services*

If casualty conscious:

1 **Stop the activity:**

- help casualty into comfortable position—usually sitting upright and leaning forward
- assess severity of attack
- check personal Action Plan (if available).

2 **Help with administration of casualty's medication:**

- give 4 puffs of a blue reliever inhaler—casualty takes a breath with each puff

  OR

  if using a spacer—casualty takes 4 breaths after each puff
- wait 4 minutes
- if no improvement, give another 4 separate puffs.

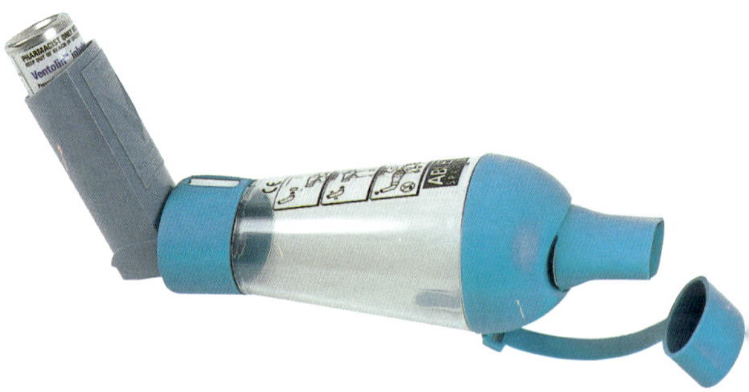

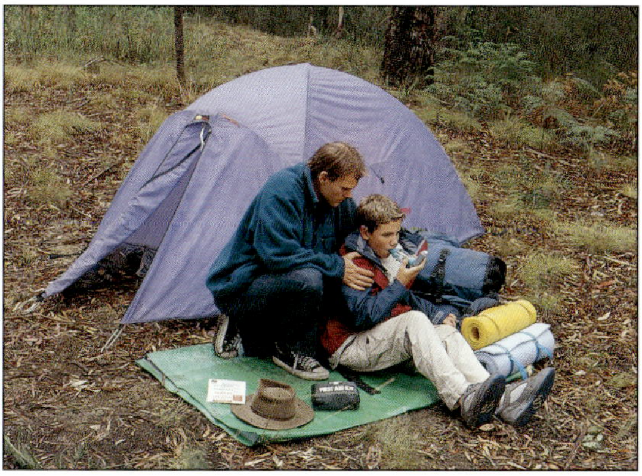

3 **If attack continues:**

- give 12 separate puffs of blue reliever inhaler
- wait 20 minutes
- if no improvement, give another 12 separate puffs.

4 **Consider evacuation of casualty if:**

- no improvement in 20 minutes after second set of 12 puffs

  OR

- reliever is required within 2 hours of the original episode.

Ongoing asthma management until help arrives or casualty is evacuated:

Casualty with mild distress may:

- be mildly anxious
- have annoying cough
- have slight increase in normal chest movement
- be able to speaks in sentences
- wheeze
- be alert

Give 4 separate puffs every hour.

Casualty with moderate distress may:

- be distressed and anxious
- show increased effort breathing and some use of neck muscles
- speak only in short phrases
- have loud wheeze
- have altered conscious state

Give 12 separate puffs every hour.

Casualty with severe distress may:

- be distressed, anxious, fighting to breathe
- be exhausted
- be confused
- show marked effort breathing
- have blue lips and be pale, sweating
- speak in single words only or be unable to speak
- have no wheeze
- have altered conscious state or be unconscious

Give 12 separate puffs every 20 minutes.

Diabetic emergency

If casualty unconscious:

- follow DRABC
- *Call Emergency Services*

If casualty conscious, and signs suggest low blood sugar:

- give sweet food or drink (not diet, diabetic or sugar-free drinks) every 15 minutes until casualty recovers or medical aid arrives
- *Call Emergency Services*

If casualty conscious, and signs suggest high blood sugar:

- allow casualty to self-administer insulin—do not administer but assist if required
- *Call Emergency Services*
- give casualty sugar-free fluids to drink, if help delayed

Note: If you are not sure which form of diabetic emergency the casualty has, give a sweet drink. If casualty has a high blood sugar emergency, then giving a sweet drink will not do undue harm.

SIGNS & SYMPTOMS

Low blood sugar

- pale
- hungry
- sweating
- weak
- confused
- aggressive

High blood sugar

- thirsty
- needs to urinate
- hot dry skin
- smell of acetone on breath

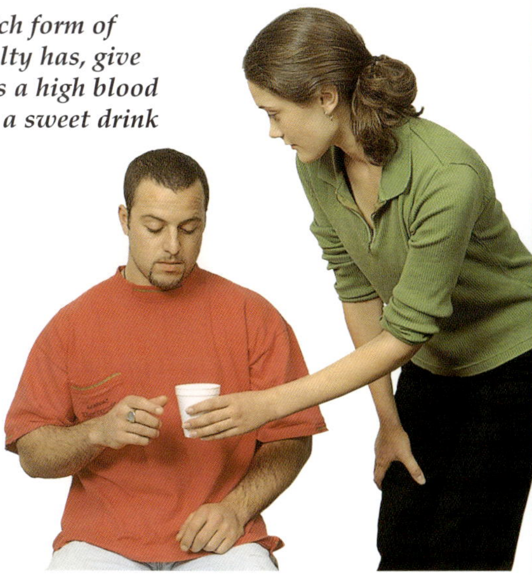

WARNING—SNAKEBITE

DO NOT wash venom off the skin.

DO NOT cut bitten area or try to suck venom out of wound.

DO NOT use a constrictive bandage.

DO NOT try to catch the snake.

Bites and stings

Snake, funnel-web spider, blue-ringed octopus, cone shell; severe allergic reaction to a bite/sting

1 **Follow DRABC.**

2 **Lie casualty down.**

3 **Reassure casualty.**

4 **Apply pressure immobilisation bandage:**

- apply crepe, elastic or other support bandage firmly—as for a sprain
- bandage from just above the fingers or toes up the limb as far as possible
- check circulation in fingers or toes.

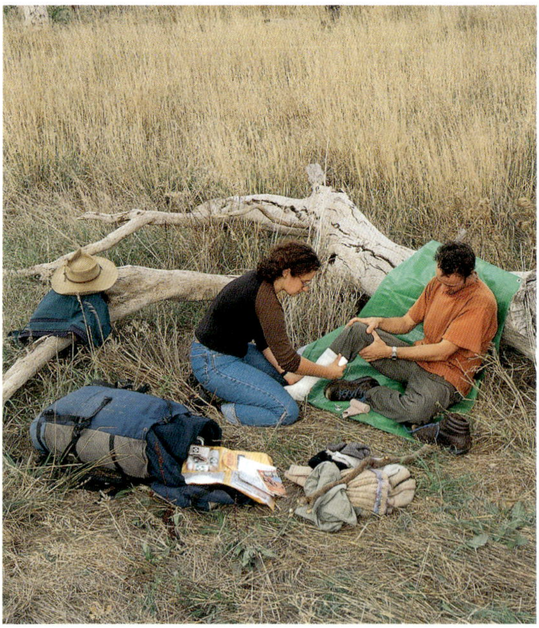

5 **Immobilise the limb by:**

- splinting—as for a fracture

OR

- bandaging arm to body or a leg to other leg.

6 *Call Emergency Services.*

7 **Keep casualty at rest:**

- if possible ensure casualty does not move
- bring help to the casualty
- continually reassure.

WARNING

Continually observe casualty's breathing—an allergic reaction can cause breathing difficulties. If casualty is unable to breathe effectively, give EAR—prepare to give CPR if required.

In addition to immobilisation, for:

Blue-ringed octopus bite:

- bites can be fatal, due to paralytic effects of venom
- effects of venom will eventually wear off—DO NOT stop EAR/ CPR until Emergency Services arrive

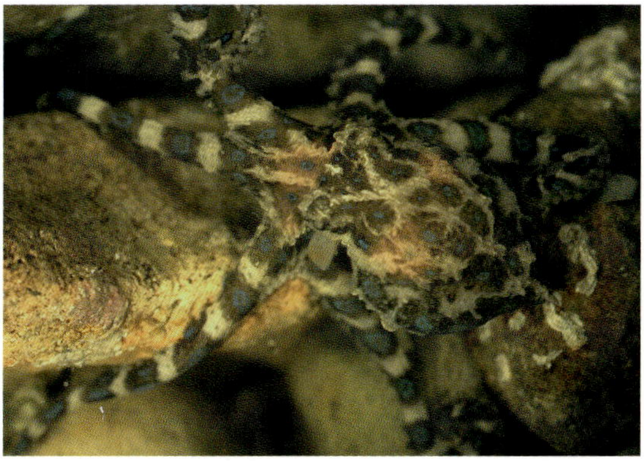

Allergic reaction:

- remove a sting if present
- *Call Emergency Services*
- if casualty has medication for allergies, it should be taken immediately
- asthma reliever medication may assist a casualty who has difficulty breathing *(see p. 152)*

Box jellyfish

The box jellyfish is extremely dangerous. It is found around the northern coast of Australia from Bundaberg on the east coast to Geraldton on the west.

1 **Do not become enmeshed in tentacles.**

2 **Flood the entire stung area with vinegar for at least 30 seconds.**

3 **Apply pressure immobilisation bandage:**
   - but NOT over stings untreated with vinegar.

4 **Immobilise the limb by:**
   - Splinting the bandaged limb
   - Ensuring casualty does not move.

5 *Call Emergency Services.*

Note: Observe safety warning signs.

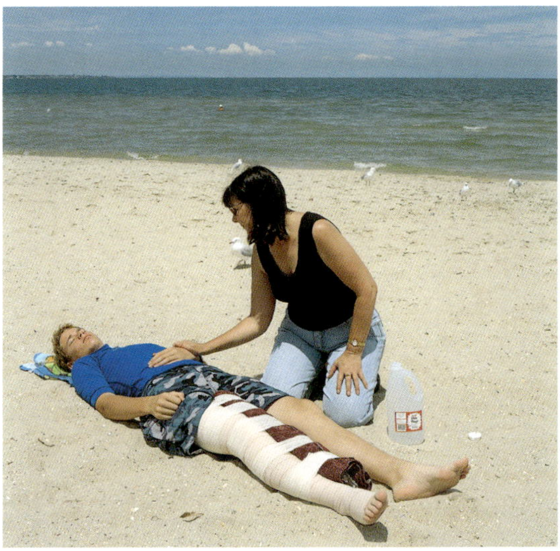

Stingray, stonefish, cobbler

1 **Observe breathing—start EAR if required.**

2 **Gently remove the barb if visible.**

3 **Immerse affected area in hot water:**

- check water temperature first.

4 ***Call Emergency Services if the wound is to chest or abdomen.***

Red-back spider, scorpion, centipede, wasp, bee

1 **If a bee sting—remove sting.**

2 **Reassure casualty.**

3 **Apply icepack/cold compress.**

4 **Observe for signs of allergic reaction.**

5 ***Call Emergency Services—for red-back spider bite.***

Tick

1 **Kill the tick:**

- apply insect repellent, kerosene or lighter fluid.

2 **Repeat after one minute.**

3 **When tick is dead:**

- brush off, or lever out with tweezers.

4 **If head of tick is left behind:**

- treat as you would a splinter.

5 **Apply cold compress if required to relieve any pain.**

NOTE

Ticks attach themselves to the body, usually in skin crevices, behind ears, in the hair or inside underwear.

Observe casualty carefully for at least 24 hours following a tick bite, monitor ABC—give CPR if required.

NOTE

Call Emergency Services if:

- level of consciousness declines
- shivering stops
- pulse is difficult to find

On recognising that a person in the group is affected by the cold, ensure everyone else is wearing wind/waterproof clothing and a hat.

Signs & symptoms

When body temperature falls, early warning signs may include:

- feeling cold, shivering
- clumsiness and slurred speech
- confusion and emotional distress
- cold/numb/blue extremities

Hypothermia

1 **Stop activity:**
   - get into shelter e.g. tent, swag or tarpaulin bag.

2 **Dry casualty:**
   - remove wet clothes
   - handle casualty gently
   - assist to put on warm dry clothing.

3 **Avoid excess activity or movement.**

4 **Warm casualty:**
   - place in sleeping-bag, or wrap in blanket
   - wrap in space blanket (only with other forms of insulation)
   - insulate from ground
   - cover head to maintain body heat.

5 **Give warm drinks and something to eat:**
   - no alcohol.

6 **Rest casualty:**
   - consider need to move in relation to casualty's recovery.

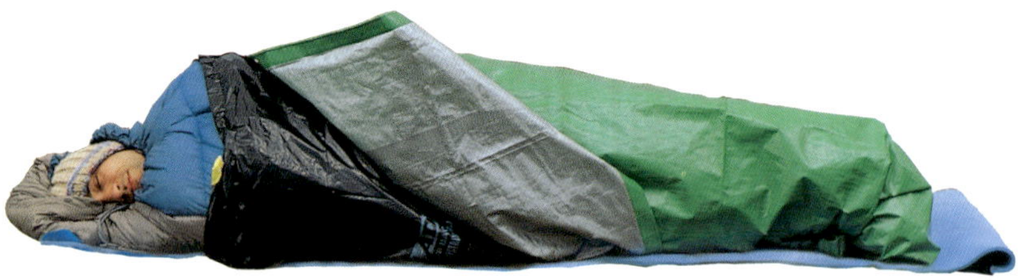

Heat-induced conditions

Heat exhaustion

1 **Lie casualty down:**

- move casualty to lie down in a cool place with circulating air.

2 **Loosen tight clothing:**

- remove unnecessary garments.

3 **Sponge with cool water and fan.**

4 **Give fluids to drink.**

5 *Call Emergency Services if:*

- casualty vomits fluids consumed, or cannot drink.

Heatstroke

1 **Rest in a cool place.**

2 **Remove excess clothing.**

3 **Apply cold packs or ice:**

- to neck, groin and armpits

OR

- if no icepack available, cover with wet towels and fan to cool.

4 *Call Emergency Services.*

SIGNS & SYMPTOMS

- feeling hot, exhausted and weak
- persistent headache
- thirst and nausea
- giddiness and faintness
- fatigue
- rapid breathing and shortness of breath
- pale, cool, clammy skin
- rapid, weak pulse

Additional symptoms

- high body temperature
- flushed skin
- irritability and mental confusion may progress to seizure and unconsciousness

WARNING

Heatstroke is a potentially fatal condition and requires urgent medical attention.

WARNING

Burns to face, hands, feet or genitals should be managed as serious burns.

If burn is large or deep, manage casualty for shock.

A casualty with extensive burns can lose a great deal of body fluid.

If casualty conscious and help is delayed, give small frequent drinks of water, until help arrives.

DO NOT apply lotions, ointment or fat to a burn.

DO NOT touch the injured areas or burst any blisters.

DO NOT remove anything sticking to the burn.

Burns

1 **Remove casualty from danger:**

- follow DRABC.

2 **If clothing on fire—STOP, DROP and ROLL:**

- pull casualty to ground
- wrap in a woollen blanket or similar, and/or roll casualty along ground until flames extinguished.

3 **Cool the burnt area:**

- hold burnt area under cold running water (not iced) until burnt area returns to normal temperature—may take some time with larger burns
- apply cold compresses—useful for burns to face and neck.

4 **Remove any constrictions:**

- remove clothing and jewellery from burnt area—unless sticking to the burn.

5 **Cover burn:**

- place sterile non-stick dressing, closely woven material over burn, e.g. triangular bandage or gladwrap.

6 **Except for very small burns, seek medical advice.**

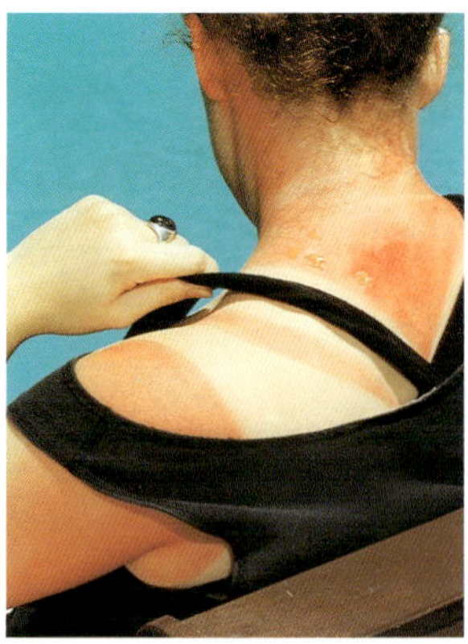

Head injury

1 **Monitor breathing and pulse:**
- if casualty unconscious, follow DRABC
- keep casualty's airway open with fingers (if face badly injured).

2 **Support head and neck:**
- support casualty's head and neck during movement in case the spine is injured.

3 **Control bleeding:**
- place sterile pad or dressing over wound
- apply direct pressure to wound unless you suspect a skull fracture
- if blood or fluid comes from ear, secure a sterile dressing lightly in place and allow to drain.

4 **Lie casualty down:**
- place casualty in comfortable position with head and shoulders slightly raised
- be prepared to turn casualty onto side if they vomit
- clear the airway quickly after vomiting.

5 ***Call Emergency Services.***

SIGNS & SYMPTOMS

- altered or abnormal responses to commands and touch
- wounds to the scalp or face
- blood or clear fluid escaping from nose or ears
- pupils becoming unequal in size
- blurred vision
- loss of memory

WARNING

Consider the possibility of a spinal injury—stabilise head and neck as soon as possible.

WARNING

DO NOT touch the eye or any contact lens.

DO NOT allow casualty to rub eye.

DO NOT try to remove any object embedded in the eye.

DO NOT apply pressure when bandaging the eye.

Eye injury

1 **Support casualty's head:**
- keep casualty's head as still as possible
- ask casualty to try not to move eyes.

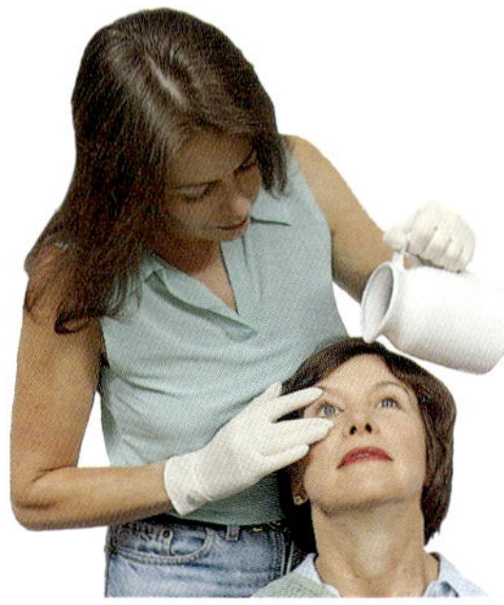

2 **Flush eye with cool, flowing water:**
- if chemical or heat burn, or smoke in eyes, flush with water.

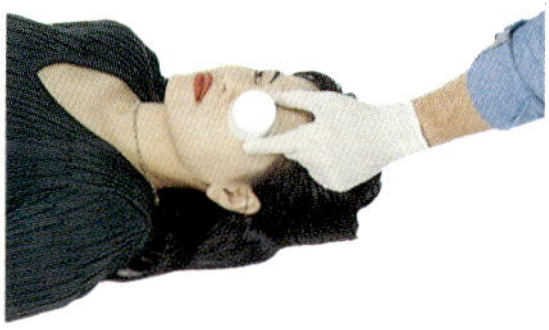

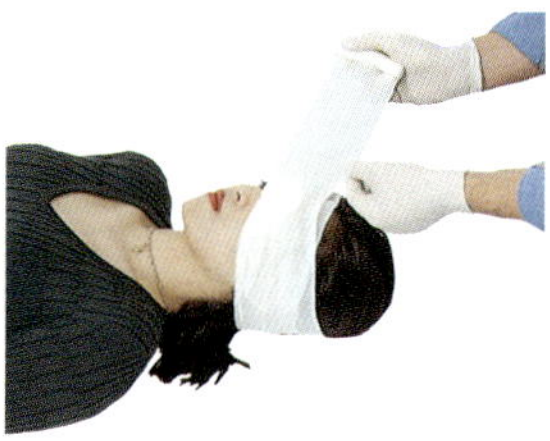

3 **Place dressing over eye:**
- place a sterile pad or dressing over injured eye
- ask casualty to hold this in place
- bandage dressing in place, covering injured eye
- if embedded object in eye, lie casualty on back, place pad around object and bandage in place.

4 ***Call Emergency Services.***

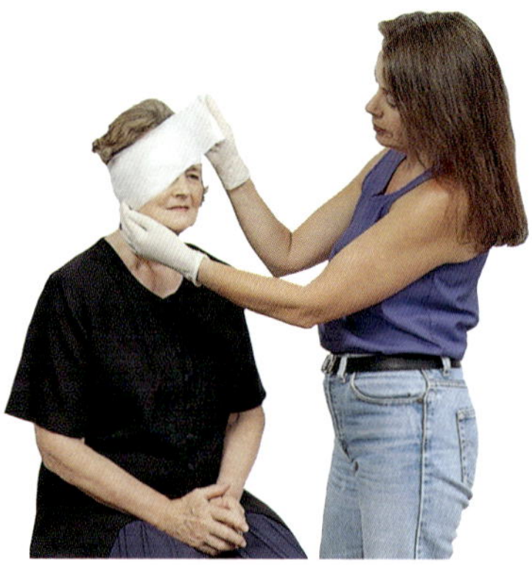

Fractures

1 **Control any bleeding and cover wounds.**

2 **If possible, manage casualty and support limb in position found.**

3 **If the limb extremity is cool, pale or blue, circulation may be reduced:**

- realignment of limb to regain circulation must be considered.

4 **Ask casualty not to move injured part.**

5 **Immobilise the fracture:**

- until it is necessary to move casualty, limb can be supported by using clothing or equipment packed on both sides of limb
- if casualty needs to be moved, use broad bandages to prevent movement at joints above and below the fracture *(see p. 103 for improvised materials)*
- support limb, carefully passing bandages under natural hollows
- place a padded splint along injured limb and pad hollows between splint and contours of limb and secure firmly *(see p. 103 for improvised splints)*
- check that bandages are not too tight or too loose every 15 minutes.

6 *Call Emergency Services.*

Note: If a leg is fractured and both legs are secured to splint, immobilise both feet and ankles with figure of eight bandage. If help is delayed, splinting the fractured leg alone may be more appropriate—immobilise one foot and ankle with the splint using a figure of eight bandage.

SIGNS & SYMPTOMS

- pain at or near site of injury
- difficult or impossible normal movement
- loss of power
- deformity or abnormal mobility
- tenderness
- swelling
- discolouration and bruising

Note

Ongoing observation:

- observe casualty for signs of shock
- check limb frequently to ensure that swelling has not caused bandages or clothing to become too tight
- check that bandages holding splint in place have not loosened with time
- pressure area care
- hygiene

NOTE

If pain is severe or deformity is present a fracture must be suspected.

It can be difficult to tell whether the injury is a fracture, dislocation, sprain or strain. If in doubt, always manage as a fracture.

If a dislocation of a joint is suspected, rest, elevate and apply ice or cold compress to joint.

If a collarbone fracture is suspected, support arm on injured side in a St John sling—a sling that supports the weight of the arm with fingers pointing to the opposite shoulder.

Sprains

1 **Rest casualty.**

2 **Elevate affected part:**

- sit with ankle resting on a pack.

3 **Remove footwear:**

- observe injury site.

4 **Apply icepack for 15 minutes every 2 hours:**

- if ice is not available, immerse part in cold water

OR

- apply a cold compress.

5 **Bandage joint firmly:**

- check regularly to ensure it is not too tight.

6 ***Emergency Services may be needed to evacuate the casualty.***

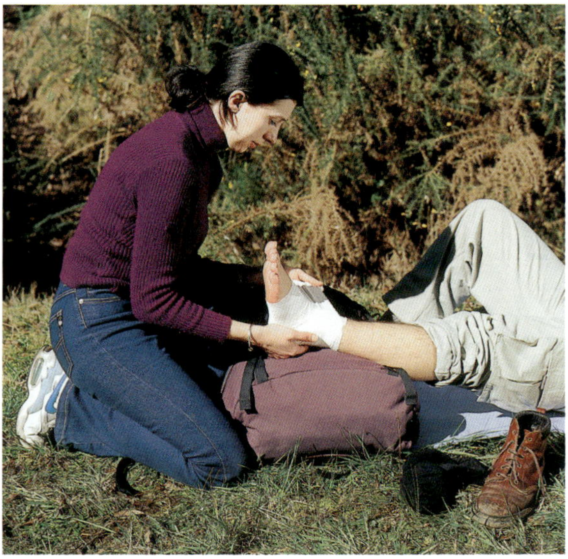

Emergency childbirth

Faced with a situation where a pregnant woman is saying that the baby is coming, it is advisable to believe her and begin making preparations for the birth.

1 **Consider the woman's privacy:**

- direct those not assisting to move away.

2 **Lie woman down:**

- on a blanket, sheet or towel.

3 **Prepare for delivery:**

- have a clean towel, pillowcase or similar available to dry off the baby
- have a clean towel available to use as a pad following the delivery of the afterbirth.

4 **Wash your hands:**

- wear gloves if available.

Note: The delivery may occur quickly or may take some considerable time. When the interval between contractions shortens and the contractions become more intense, the process of delivery has begun.

5 **Position yourself so that you can assist the baby as it is being delivered.**

6 **Encourage the woman to pant and not to hold her breath.**

7 **As the baby's head appears:**

- be prepared to support its head and body in your hands.

8 **Do not pull the baby.**

9 As soon as the baby is born:

- lay it on a clean sheet or towel between the mother's legs
- dry it off quickly
- wrap it in a clean towel or sheet to keep warm.

10 By this stage, most babies are either crying or making some noise; if not:

- gently open the baby's mouth and check that there is not fluid remaining in the mouth; if necessary, clear the baby's mouth of fluid.

11 Place baby on mother's abdomen:

- don't pull on the umbilical cord.

12 Shortly after birth of baby, afterbirth will be delivered.

13 Place a sanitary pad in position and massage mother's lower abdomen:

- this will help to reduce excessive bleeding.

14 Leave afterbirth attached to the baby:

- place afterbirth in a suitable container for protection.

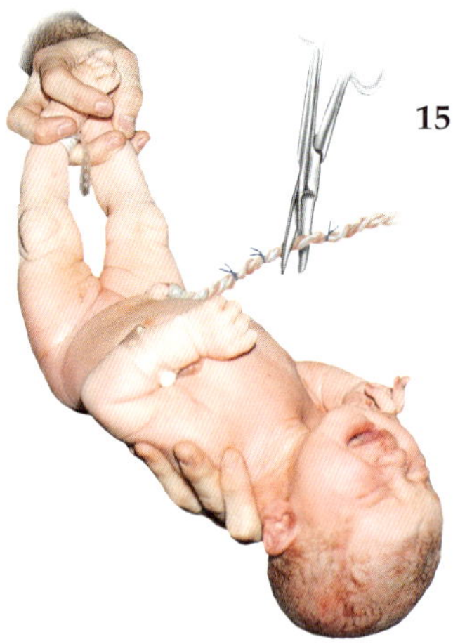

15 If the arrival of medical help is going to take an excessively long time, cut umbilical cord as follows:

- firmly tie with sterile string in 3 places—10 cm, 15 cm, and 20 cm from baby's navel to prevent bleeding after it is cut
- cut between 2nd and 3rd tie away from baby
- cover stump of cord loosely with a sterile dressing
- check cord for bleeding every 15 minutes for first hour then half hourly until Emergency Services arrive.

Glossary

Acute phase initial first aid management to control a life-threatening situation

Adrenaline (epinephrine) a hormone that occurs naturally in the body; when given by injection, it relaxes constricted airways

Allergic reaction reaction in some people caused by contact with a substance foreign to the body such as bee venom or certain foods

Analgesic a drug that relieves pain

Antenna a radio aerial

Antibiotics prescribed medication used for the management of infections

Antidiarrhoeics drug or agent that relieves the symptoms of diarrhoea

Antifungal a substance that kills fungi or inhibits their growth or reproduction

Antihistamines substance used to manage allergies

Antiseptic a substance that kills or prevents the growth of disease-causing bacteria

APIE assess, plan, implement, evaluate—cyclical management plan

Assessment evaluation of problems affecting casualty as indicated by history, symptoms and signs observed by first aider

Asthma spasm of bronchial (breathing) tubes in the lungs

Bearing the direction of an object from an observer, measured in degrees relative to true or magnetic north

Blizzard a severe snowstorm

Cardiac relating to heart

Cardiopulmonary resuscitation (CPR) resuscitation technique that combines expired air resuscitation (EAR) with external cardiac compressions (ECC)

Casualty a person, alive or dead, who has suffered an injury or sudden illness

CB citizens' band radio

Cervical collar (neck collar) used to support the neck

Chafing superficial irritation of the skin caused by friction

Chlorine tablet used to purify water, e.g. Puratabs

Circulation movement of blood through body

Coaxial cable consists of two concentric conductors separated by an insulator

Compass instrument showing the direction of magnetic north and bearings relative to north

Contaminated waste material containing body fluids that have the potential to be infectious

Contingency plan a plan to cope with unforeseen circumstances

CPR cardiopulmonary resuscitation

Dehydration excessive loss of water from body

Diabetes disease caused by loss of insulin-producing cells in pancreas, or by decreased insulin production or functioning

Diarrhoea overly frequent and soft or liquid bowel motions

DRABC Danger, Response, Airway, Breathing, Circulation—St John universal action plan for first aid management

Dressing material used to cover a wound

EAR expired air resuscitation

ECC external cardiac compressions

Electromagnetic forces forces set up by a difference of potential in an electric field

EPIRB Emergency Position Indicating Radio Beacon

Expired air resuscitation (EAR) mouth-to-mouth or mouth-to-nose-and-mouth resuscitation technique used when casualty is unable to breathe

Faeces waste products of digestion passed by the bowel

Faraday cage a wire mesh cage used to shield sensitive electronic equipment from stray radio emissions

Flares flame or bright light used as a signal

Fracture a break in a bone

Freeze-dried frozen and dried by evaporation of moisture in a high vacuum

Fungal infection any inflammatory condition caused by fungus

Gas gangrene the death of tissue cells accompanied by gas bubbles after trauma

GPS Global Positioning System used for navigation; radio signals are sent to and from satellites to determine a position on the ground

Grid reference a position on a map given in relation to the grid lines on the map

HF high frequency radio

HIV (human immunodeficiency virus) causes clinical illness called AIDS

Hypothermia excessive cooling of the body, usually accidental and often serious

Infection invasion and growth of harmful germs in tissues and fluids of body

Iodine tablet used to purify water

IV equipment used in intravenous therapy

Line of sight the straight line along which an observer looks

Medication medicine in any form—liquid, tablet, inhalant or injected substance

Nausea a feeling of sickness with possible vomiting

Neck collar (cervical collar) used to support the neck

Oxygen a life-sustaining gaseous element of air

Povidine Iodine an antiseptic for disinfecting wounds Pressure pad firm pad applied over dressing to assist in control of bleeding

Pressure points the points where arteries lie over bones and hence where pressure can be applied to control bleeding

Protractor instrument for measuring angles, usually a semicircle marked off in degrees

Puffer (inhaler) device to deliver a regulated dose of asthma medication

Pulse transmission of heartbeat felt in various parts of the body

Pupil opening in centre of iris (coloured part) of eye

Rehydration restoration of normal water balance by giving fluids

Response a casualty's reply to a first aider's 'shake and shout', enabling assessment of casualty's state of consciousness

RFDS Royal Flying Doctor Service; a remote area medical service in Australia

Salbutamol used as a bronchodilator in the management of an asthma attack

Saline a clear solution containing sodium chloride generally used for flushing loose debris from eyes and cleaning wounds

Satellite phone a phone that uses satellites for the communication link

Shock a condition in which the circulatory system is not carrying sufficient blood to the tissues

SOS international code-signal of extreme distress, an urgent appeal for help

Spacer device to improve delivery of asthma medication by a puffer/inhaler

Sprain stretching of ligaments beyond their normal range

Sterilisation tablets tablets used to purify water, e.g. chlorine or iodine tablets

Strain overstretching or overexertion of a muscle

Symptoms what casualty tells you about his or her condition

Taint an unpleasant taste in water

Taxiing of an aircraft—to go along the ground surface under the machine's own power before or after flying

Tetanus serious and potentially fatal infection, characterised by muscle spasms

Thermorest™ trademark for a thin mattress that insulates from the ground

Tinea fungus infection of skin

Trauma wound, injury or other shocking experience

UHF ultra-high frequency radio

Umbilical cord attaches unborn baby to placenta in mother's uterus

Venom a toxin (i.e. a poison made by a living thing), usually from a snake, insect, spider or marine creature; injected by bite or sting

Vomiting reflex action causing stomach contents to be ejected through mouth

Water bladder soft sac or bag that holds liquid

Water vessel hollow structure designed to travel on water and carry people and/or goods

Wheel ruts ridges in the ground caused by a vehicle on soft ground

Wind chill factor apparent temperature drop perceived by the exposed skin caused by the wind

Windsock canvas cylinder or cone on a mast which indicates the direction of the wind

Index

St John Ambulance Australia

St John Ambulance Australia is a self-funding, charitable organisation, active in every State and Territory, dedicated to helping people in sickness, distress, suffering or danger.

We have been active in Australia for over one hundred years, and are part of a wider international organisation with a long and honourable history.

Our uniformed volunteers in their familiar black and white uniforms provide the highest quality first aid coverage at sport and community events.

Non-uniformed volunteers support the vulnerable in need of friendship, compassionate care or a little help.

In Western Australia and the Northern Territory we run the public ambulance service. Paid and volunteer ambulance officers provide critical response and non-emergency patient transport.

St John Volunteers also support crucial fundraising and awareness programs.

St John is a self-funding charity: we do not rely on Government funding.

St John is Australia's largest first aid trainer, teaching practical life-saving skills to around a quarter of a million people each year. Our courses are designed to accommodate all aspects of first aid training. Courses can also be designed to meet specific industry needs.

One of the courses conducted by St John is Remote Area First Aid which is designed for people who travel or work in remote areas, are completing an outdoor education course, or like to go kayaking, hiking, canoeing, four wheel driving or skiing; to name but a few activities. This course will help you prepare for your activity and teach you how to manage emergency situations, including evacuations; and much more.

As a companion to the remote area first aid course, this book doubles as a tool for both planning your activity and, should the occasion arise, as a reference to first aid management in remote areas of Australia when help is hours or even days away.

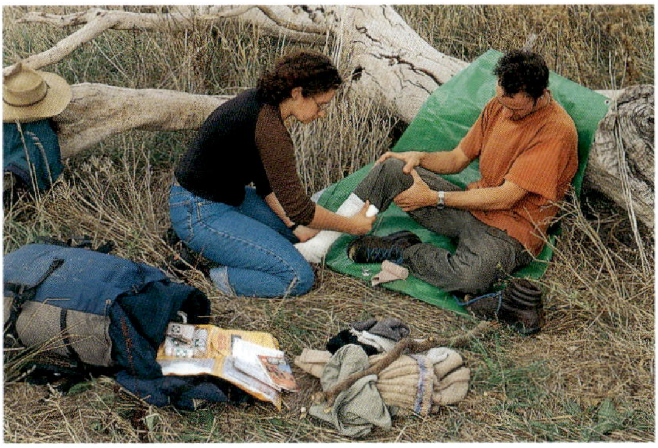

St John also provides a comprehensive range of first aid kits and products for the home, workplace, car, boat or holiday. Among our range of kits are those specifically designed for use in a remote area. These first aid kits contain contents and specific packaging required to cater for activities normally carried out in remote areas.

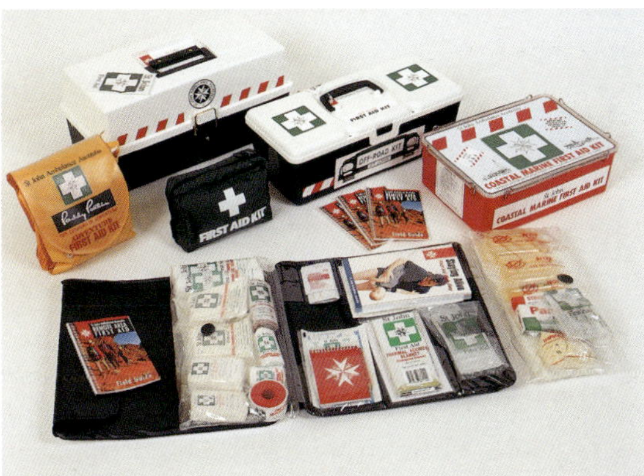

To find out more about first aid training courses, first aid kits and equipment, or becoming a volunteer member of St John Ambulance Australia contact St John in your State or Territory, toll free on 1300 360 455 or visit our web site, www.stjohn.org.au.

Notes